FOOD
Recipes

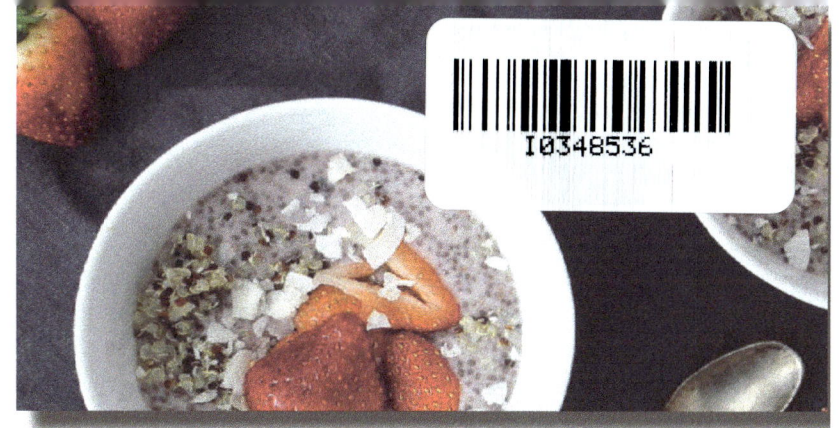

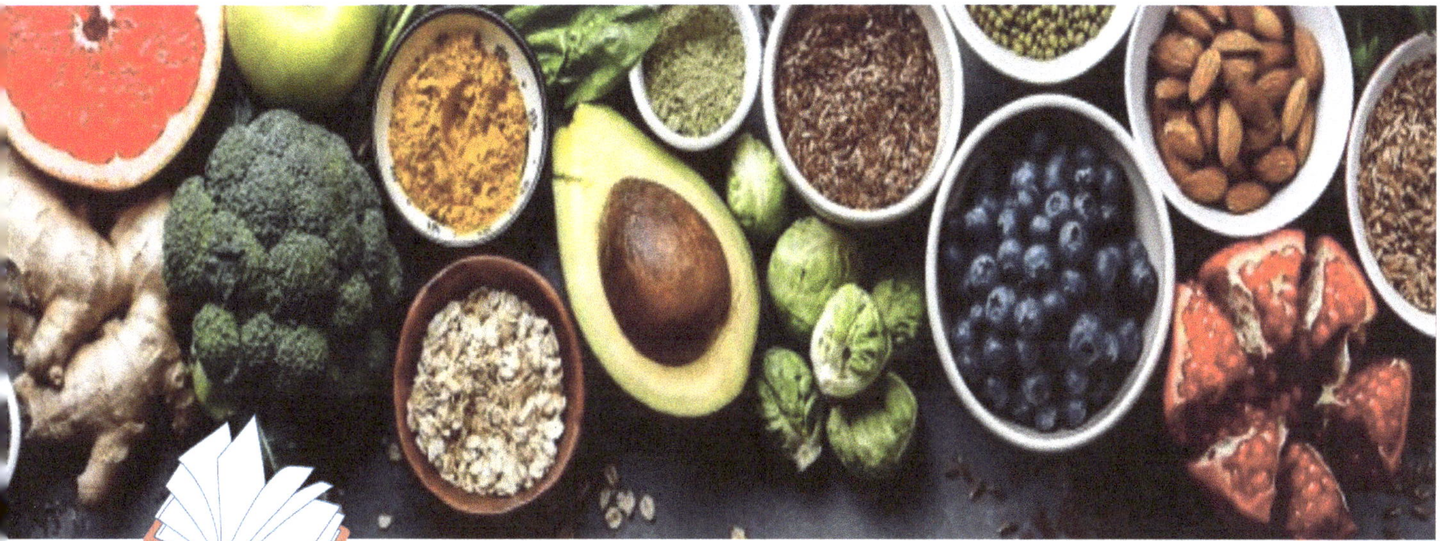

By
S.MARIE

ALKALINE LIFE

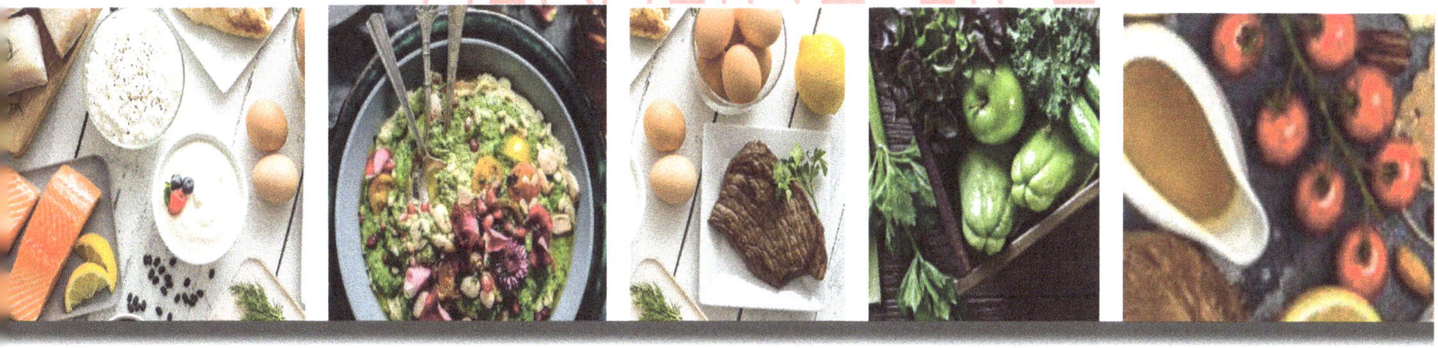

WWW.ALKALINELIFE.SHOP

copyright © 2024 by Discovering Solutions
Author: Sheena Marie

All rights reserved. No part of this publication may be reproduced, distributed or trans-mitted in any form or by any means, including photocopying, recording, or other elec-tronic or mechanical methods, without the prior written permission of the publisher, except in the case of brief quotations embodied in critical reviews and certain other noncommercial uses permitted by copyright law.

Library of Congress Control Number: 2024944683
Discovering Solutions
https://www.discoverings.biz
Book Design : Cover Design / Discovering Solutions.
ISBN 978-1-7324187-8-3

TABLE OF CONTENT

SPROUTED ALMOND BUTTER	05
ALMOND MILK AND ALMOND PULP CHEESE	07
STRAWBERRY AND SPINACH SUPER SMOOTHIE	09
BLUEBERRY DELIGHT ALKALINE SMOOTHIE	10
STRAWBERRY COCO CHIA QUINOA BREAKFAST	11
SWEET AND SAVORY SALAD	13
NON-DAIRY APPLE PARFAIT	14
SAVORY AVOCADO WRAP	15

ALMOND BUTTER CRUNCH BERRY SMOOTHIE	16
KALE PESTO PASTA	17
APPLE AND ALMOND BUTTER OATS	18
GREEN GODDESS BOWL/AVOCADO CUMIN DRESSING	19
BERRY GOOD SPINACH POWER SMOOTHIE	21
QUINOA MORNING PORRIDGE	23
THAI QUINOA SALAD	24
WARRIOR CHIA BREAKFAST	26
ASIAN SESAME DRESSING AND NOODLES	28
FRENCH TOAST	29
APPLE PANCAKES	30
AVOCADO BREAKFAST SALAD	34

MIX SPROUT SALAD	36
KALE CHICKPEA HUMMUS	38
QUINOA AND APPLE BREAKFAST	40
EASY ALKALINE YOGURT	41
YUMMY COLD OATS	43
CRAMBLED "EGGS" (TOFU SCRAMBLE)	44
THEPLAS	46
MAPLE MILLET PORRIDGE	49
CHICKPEA FRITTATA	51
LEAN GREEN FENNEL MINT SMOOTHIE	53
ALKALINE NOT NACHOS	54
EDAMAME AND MUSHROOM PASTA	56

INTRODUCTION

The alkaline diet has become popular for its numerous health benefits. Several nutritionists believe that the modern diet is high in acidic food which may negatively impact multiple bodily functions. That is why trying out some amazing alkaline breakfast recipes may be the best way to balance the pH levels in your body. In this book, take a look at some of the simple alkaline recipes you can try from the comfort of your home.

Introducing Sheena Marie: A Beacon of Healing and Wholeness. Meet Marie isa blessed and experienced individual whose journey from illness to vitality has inspired countless others to reclaim their health and well-being. Having triumphed over malignant tumors herself, Sheena Marie's personal healing journey ignited a passion for helping others to discover the transformative power of holistic healing. Drawing upon her extensive training under luminaries such as Dr. Sebi, Samma Bowman, and Fanny Garcia, Sheena Marie has become a beacon of hope and healing in the realm of natural medicine. As a medical professional in the US, Sheena Marie combines her expertise in diet, herbal medicine, and spiritual practices to facilitate profound healing experiences for those she serves. Her dedicated efforts,

she has guided numerous individuals on their paths to recovery from various diseases and ailments, using a combination of nourishing recipes and potent herbal remedies. Her compassionate approach and unwavering commitment to holistic wellness have earned her the trust and admiration of countless souls seeking to reclaim their health and vitality. In this recipe book, Sheena Marie shares her most cherished recipes for an alkaline diet, alongside insights gleaned from her own healing journey and years of experience in natural medicine. Get ready to embark on a journey of healing and wholeness with Sheena Marie as your guide.

In your life, each meal represents a thread of love, woven with care and intention. You are the artist of your own destiny, creating a masterpiece of wellness and vitality with every bite.

SPROUTED ALMOND
BUTTER

RECIPE 01

INGREDIENTS

- 3 CUPS ALMONDS
- 1/2 TSP SALT FOR SOAKING
- 6 CUPS WATER FOR SOAKING
- 1/2 TSP SALT (OPTIONAL)

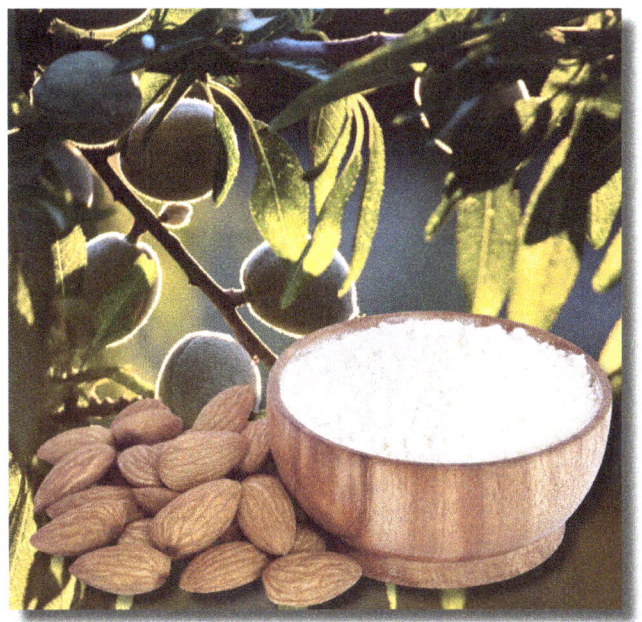

NOTES

Making your own activated almond nut butter is a fun and tasty way to get the freshest nut butter around. Suitable for raw-vegan, oil-free, paleo, gluten-free, and sugar-free diets. Full of heart healthy fats from the almonds, with no added oil.

This almond nut butter is 100% pure nuts with just a pinch of salt added. The nuts are activated meaning they are easier to digest and less likely to cause that heavy, upset-stomach feeling you can get with nuts. This nut butter recipe makes sweet, salted, almond nut butter.

If you don't have a powerful blender, add a few tablespoons of cold pressed oil once the nuts are broken down to dust. This does speed up the process and less powerful blenders may take too long or get damaged making nut butter.
Store almond butter in the fridge and enjoy within a few weeks

May these alkaline recipes be a source of inspiration and empowerment on your path to vibrant health. With each meal, you are taking a powerful step toward a brighter, healthier future.

INSTRUCTIONS

1. Soak the nuts for 8 hours or overnight with ½ tsp salt.

2. Drain and rinse, then spread out and either bake in an oven or dry in a dehydrator.

3. Oven: put the oven on the lowest temperature possible. Bake with the door ajar for 2-3 hours
until bone dry and crispy. Toss every hour.

4. Dehydrator: dry for 8-12 hours at 110F / 43C until crispy and dry. Toss halfway through.
Place the nuts in a blender or food processor while still warm and blend for 2-minute intervals.

5. Scrape the sides down between the blending sessions and repeat until a liquid almond butter is formed.

6. Add ½ tsp of salt on the final blend for salted almond butter.

In my powerful (1800W) food processor, this took about 10-12 minutes.

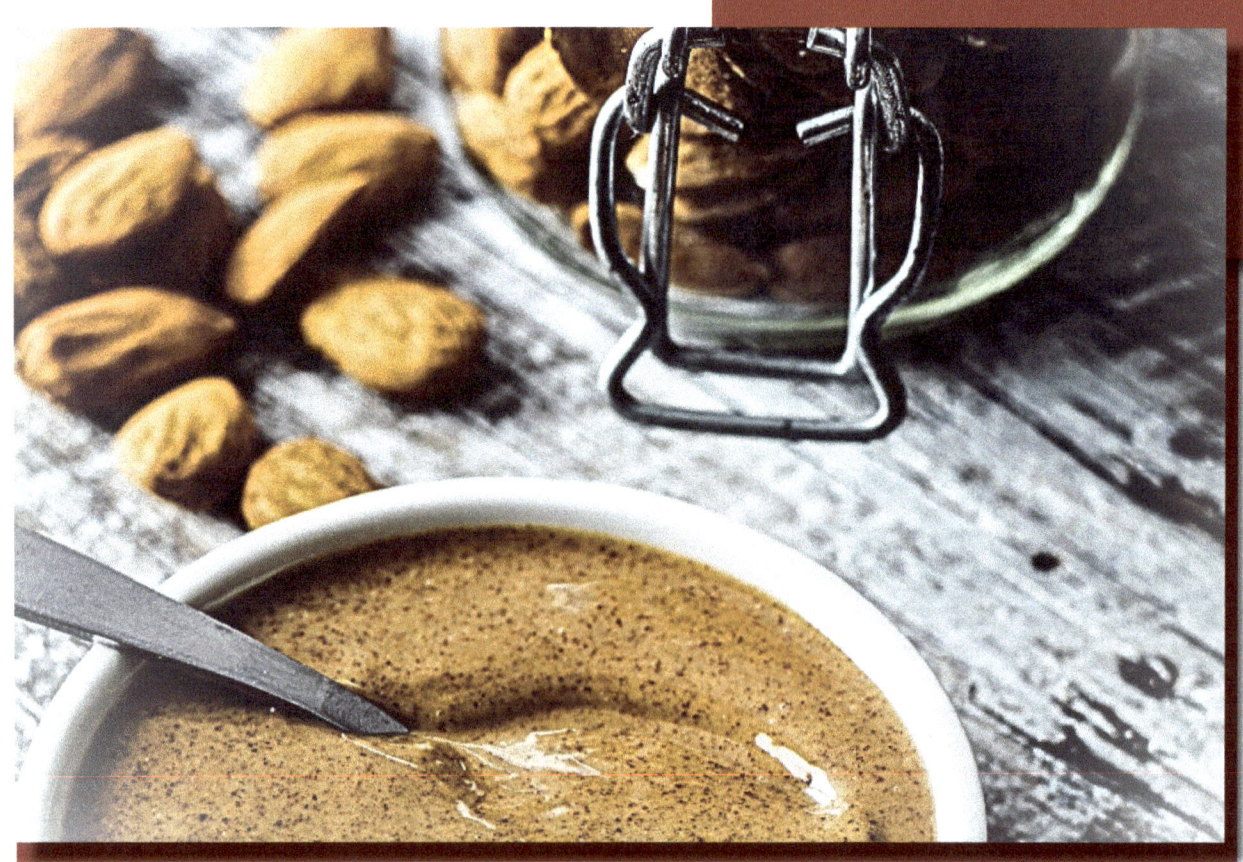

RECIPE 6 BOOK

ALMOND MILK AND PULP CHEESE

RECIPE 02

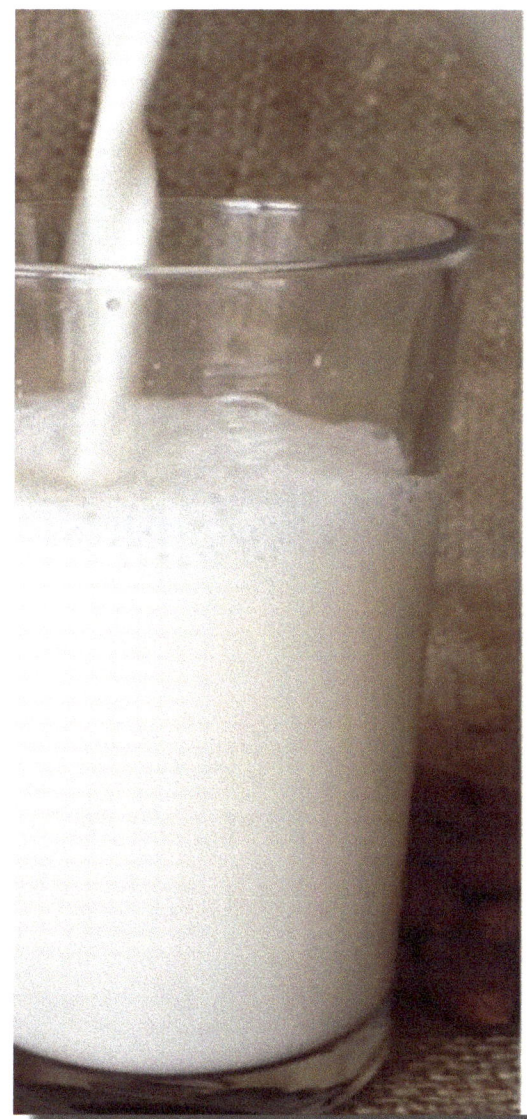
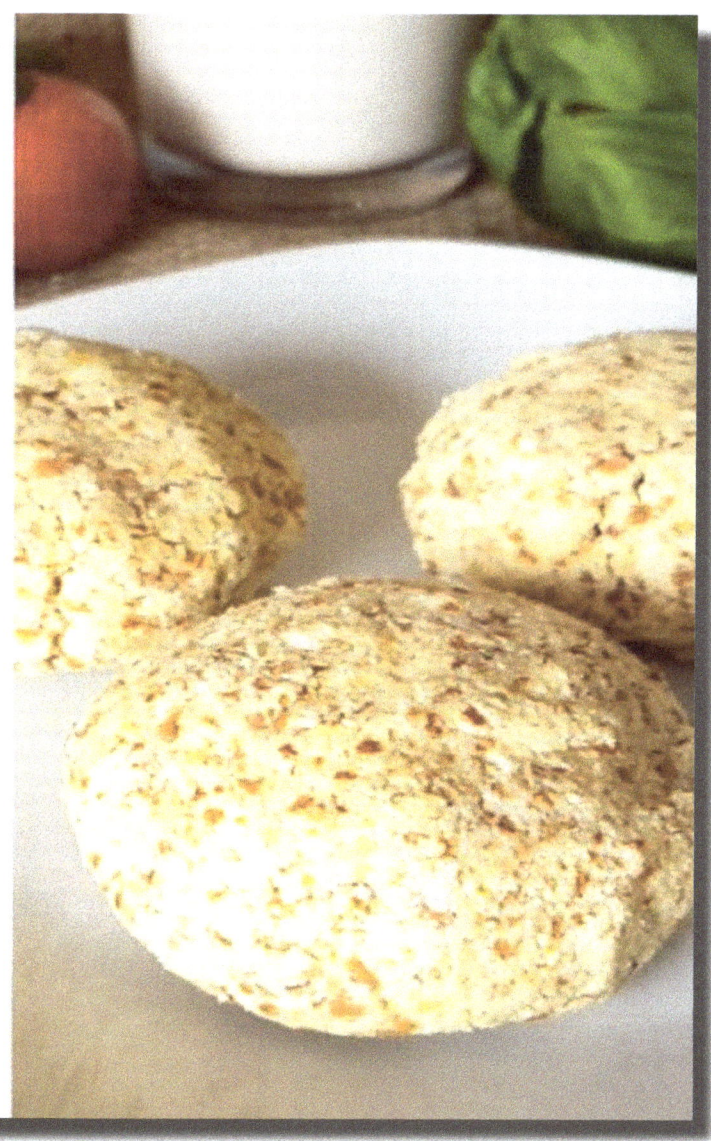

INGREDIENTS

- 1½ cups / 200g Almonds
- 4 cups Water
- 1/2 tsp Salt
- 1 tsp Vanilla
- 2 tbsp Sweetener, Maple / Date syrup or similar
- 3 tbsp Nutritional Yeast
- 1½ tbsp Coconut Oil
- 1 Lemon, juiced
- 1/2 tsp Garlic Powder
- 1/4 tsp Salt
- 1/4 tsp Powder
- 1/4 tsp Cayenne Pepper

INSTRUCTIONS

1. Soak the almonds in salted water for 8 hours or overnight to sprout them. If you are short of time, then a 1-hour soak is acceptable but less than ideal for maximum nutritional benefit.

2. Drain and rinse the almonds, then place in a blender with the fresh water.

3. Blend for a few minutes.

4. Pour into a cheesecloth/nut bag or sieve and squeeze out the almond milk. You can make your nut milk bag from some nylon if you're handy with sewing.

5. Stir in the vanilla and sweetener (date syrup) into the almond milk, if desired.

6. Empty the almond pulp into a bowl with all the other almond cheese ingredients.

7. Mix together, then roll into portion-sized cheese balls and chill.

8. The coconut oil helps to make a firm ball but can be replaced with coconut butter if you prefer.

9. Enjoy the cheese and milk within three days and store in the fridge.

10. True wellness encompasses body, mind, and spirit. With these alkaline recipes, you are nourishing your body and your entire being.

NOTES

Almond milk and almond cheese are easy to make at home. Homemade always tastes much better than shop-bought. This creamy almond milk is nutritionally superior, with a high nut content and a healthy dose of protein. The almonds are soaked and sprouted in water to aid nutrients into your body.

Make your almond milk at home that's bursting with goodness, and don't waste any pulp. With this vegan milk and cheese recipe, the almond pulp is made into a great-tasting vegan cheese with a nutty, cheesy flavor. Most almond milk from the shops is full of stabilizers, preservatives, and very few almonds. This homemade almond milk recipe is made with sprouted almonds, making it much easier for your body to absorb.

STRAWBERRY AND SPINACH SUPER **SMOOTHIE**

RECIPE 03

INGREDIENTS

2 cups Spinach

1/2 cup Strawberries

1 Lime

1 cup Coconut Water

1 tbsp Hemp Seeds

NOTES

This refreshing Strawberry and Spinach smoothie will help keep you energized throughout the day. Like blueberries, strawberries are also rich in antioxidants that help fight chronic diseases. Spinach and other leafy greens are the pillars of alkaline foods due to their high alkalinity content. Other health benefits include bone health, aiding digestion, and preventing heart diseases.
This leaves you with an excellent full but light feeling that you will embrace as you continue on this Alkalife journey.
The antioxidant properties in coconut water help reduce inflammation and prevent kidney stones.

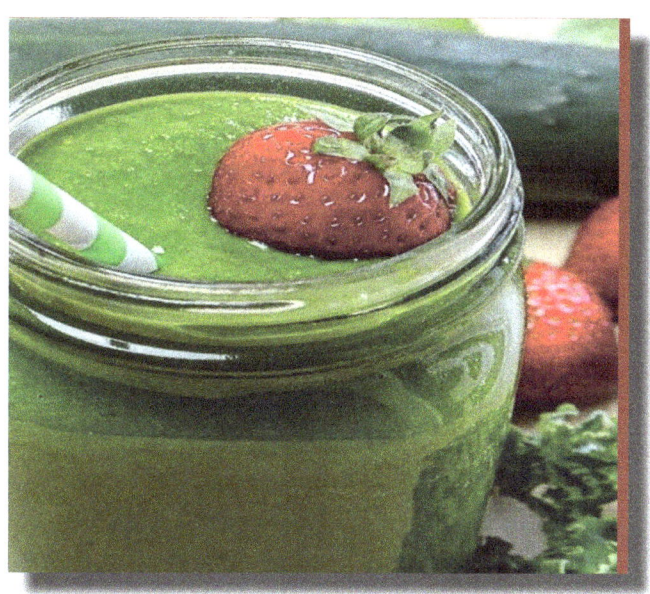

INSTRUCTIONS

1. Put all the ingredients in a blender.

2. Blend them until smooth. Note: don't place the whole lime in the blender. Instead, squeeze the 1 Lime, juiced out of it.

3. You can add some stevia to sweeten the smoothie.

4. In a world filled with fad diets and quick fixes, these alkaline recipes offer a timeless reminder of the simple power of whole, natural foods to heal and nourish..

BLUEBERRY DELIGHT ALKALINE SMOOTHIE

RECIPE 04

INGREDIENTS

1/2 cup Blueberries

1 tbsp Raw Almond Butter

1 Handful of Spinach

1 tbsp Chia Seeds

1 tbsp Ground Flax Seeds

1 cup Coconut Milk

1 tbsp Coconut Oil

1 tbsp Hemp Seed Powder

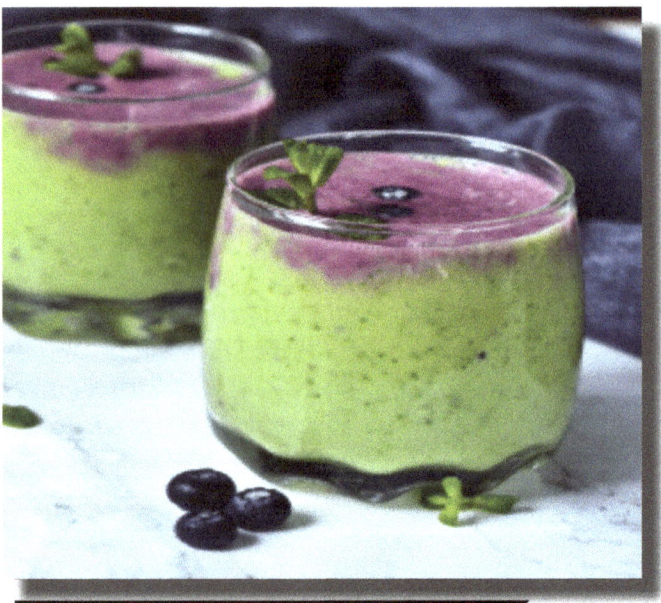

NOTES

Blueberries are great antioxidants. They are also one of the most nutrient-dense foods you can find. The antioxidants help prevent chronic diseases like heart disease, diabetes, and cancer. Blueberries make a great addition to any alkaline smoothie. This blueberry breakfast smoothie will boost your energy and keep you feeling fuller longer.

he journey to health and vitality is not always easy, but it is always worth it. With these alkaline recipes as your guide, you are well-equipped to embrace the journey with courage and grace.

INSTRUCTIONS

1. Blend the ingredients, and your smoothie will be ready. Note that you can replace the coconut milk with hemp milk, depending on your preference.

2. Serving Size: 1

STRAWBERRY COCO CHIA
QUINOA

RECIPE 05

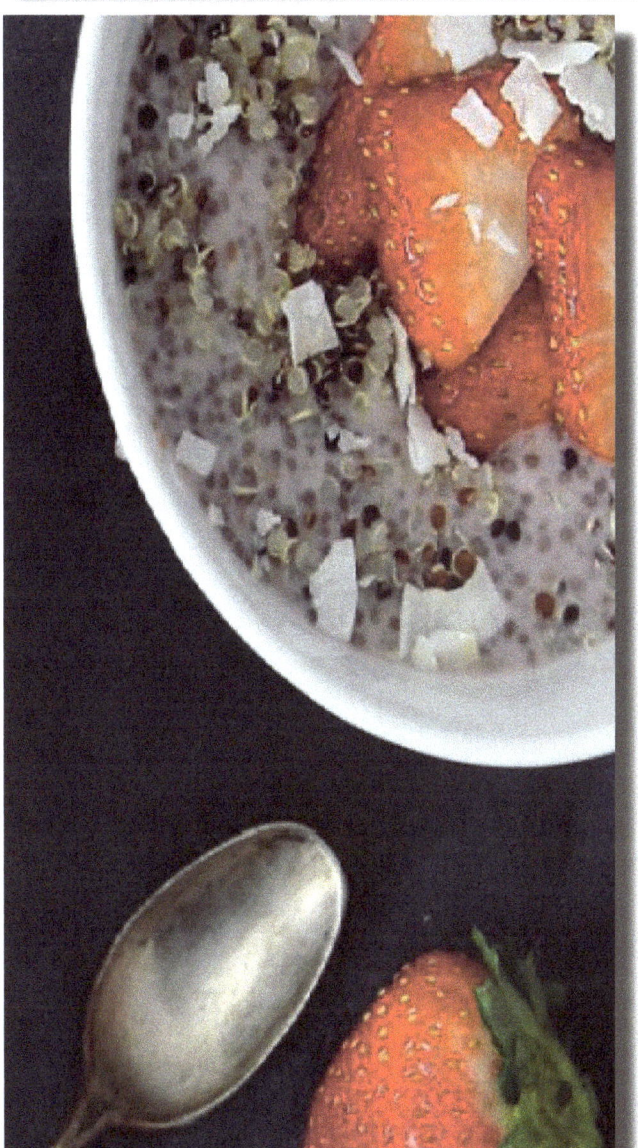

INGREDIENTS

1 cup Cooked Quinoa

5 tbsp Chia Seeds

1½ cup Almond, Coconut or Hemp Milk

1/2 cup quartered Strawberries + 4 Strawberries, sliced

2 Dates, pitted

2 tbsp Almond Pieces

2 tbsp Unsweetened Shredded Coconut Flakes

INSTRUCTIONS

1. The night before, cook quinoa and prepare strawberry chia by combining the strawberries, almond milk, and two dates in a blender and pureeing until smooth.

2. Pour the mixture into a jar and add chia seeds.

3. Mix well until all chia seeds are covered with the liquid.

4. Cover with a lid and refrigerate overnight. In the morning, place chia seeds in a bowl, add the quinoa and strawberry slices, almonds, shredded coconut, and enjoy.

NOTES

Remember that you hold the power to transform your health and your life. With each meal prepared from these alkaline recipes, you are stepping into your power and reclaiming your vitality.

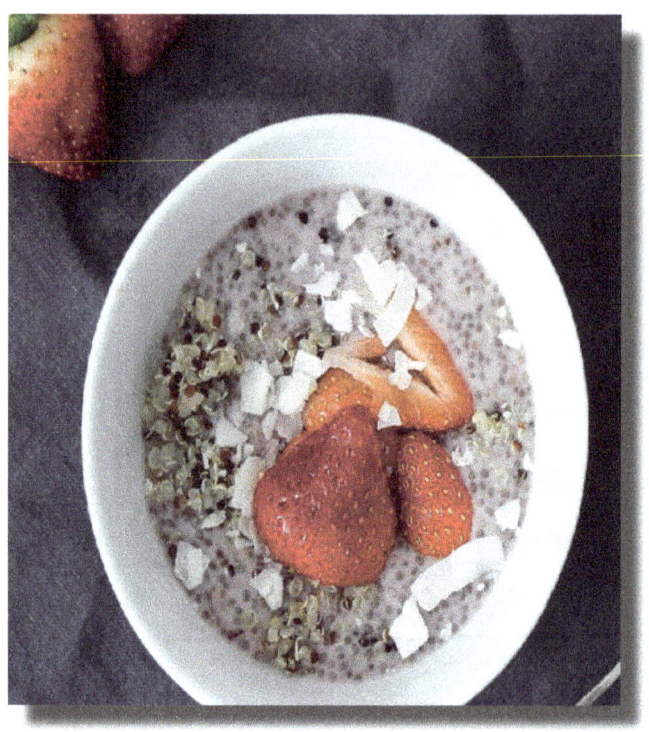

SWEET AND SAVORY
SALAD

RECIPE 06

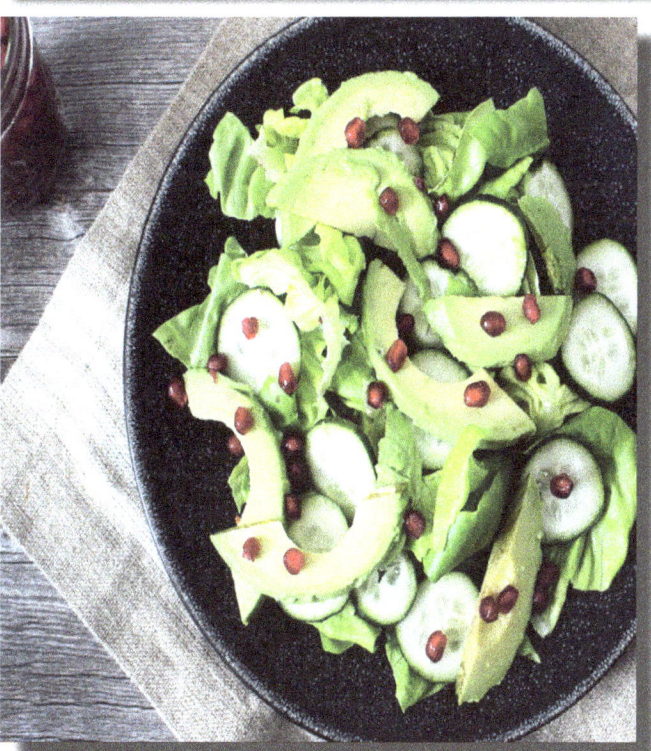

INGREDIENTS

1 Large Head of Butter Lettuce

1/2 Cucumber, sliced

1 Pomegranate, seeded, or 1/3 cup seeds

1 Avocado, cubed

1/4 cup shelled Pistachios, chopped

Dressing Ingredients:

1/4 cup Apple Cider Vinegar

1/2 cup Extra Virgin Olive Oil

1 Garlic Clove, minced

INSTRUCTIONS

1. Hand tear the butter lettuce into a salad bowl.

2. Add the rest of the ingredients and toss with the salad dressing.

NOTES

Enjoy the Blissful simple joys of life.

NON-DAIRY APPLE
PARFAIT

RECIPE 07

INGREDIENTS

1/2 cup Raw Cashews (soak 20 mins-1 hour)

1/2 cup Unsweetened Almond or Coconut Milk

1/2 tsp Vanilla

1 cup Chopped Apple

1/3 cup Rolled Gluten-Free Oats, uncooked

1 tbsp Hemp Seeds

NOTES

Remember, dear reader, that you hold the power to transform your health and your life. With each meal prepared from these alkaline recipes, you are stepping into your power and reclaiming your vitality.

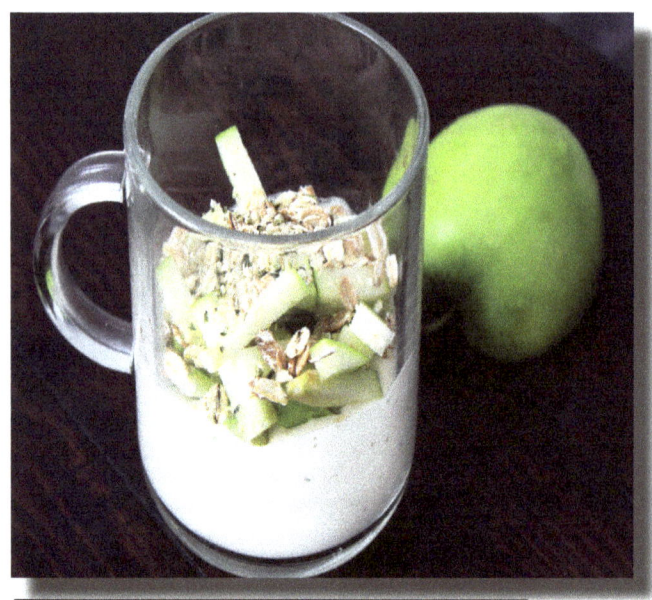

INSTRUCTIONS

1. Combine cashews, almond milk, and vanilla in a blender and blend until smooth.

2. Layer ingredients in a small cup: a heaping spoon of cashew cream, a spoonful of apples, and top with oats and hemp seeds, and enjoy.

SAVORY AVOCADO
WRAP

RECIPE 08

INGREDIENTS

1 Butter Lettuce or Collard Leaf bunch

1/2 Avocado

1 tsp Chopped Basil

Small handful of spinach

1 tsp Cilantro, chopped

1/4 cup Red Onion, diced

1 Tomato, sliced or chopped

Sea Salt and Pepper

NOTES

Your health is your greatest wealth. Invest in yourself with these alkaline recipes, and watch as your vitality and well-being flourish.

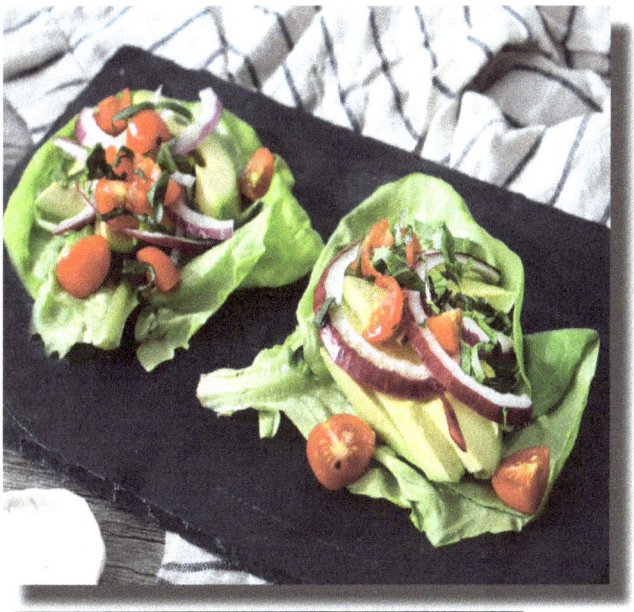

INSTRUCTIONS

1. Spread avocado onto lettuce leaf and sprinkle with basil, cilantro, red onion, tomato, salt and pepper and add spinach. Fold in half and enjoy.

ALMOND BUTTER CRUNCH BERRY SMOOTHIE

RECIPE 09

INGREDIENTS

2 cups Fresh Spinach

2 cups Almond Milk, unsweetened

1 cup of any of the following:

- frozen mixed berries, strawberries or grapes

1 Banana (peeled and frozen)

4 tbsp Raw Almond Butter

1 tbsp Chia Seeds

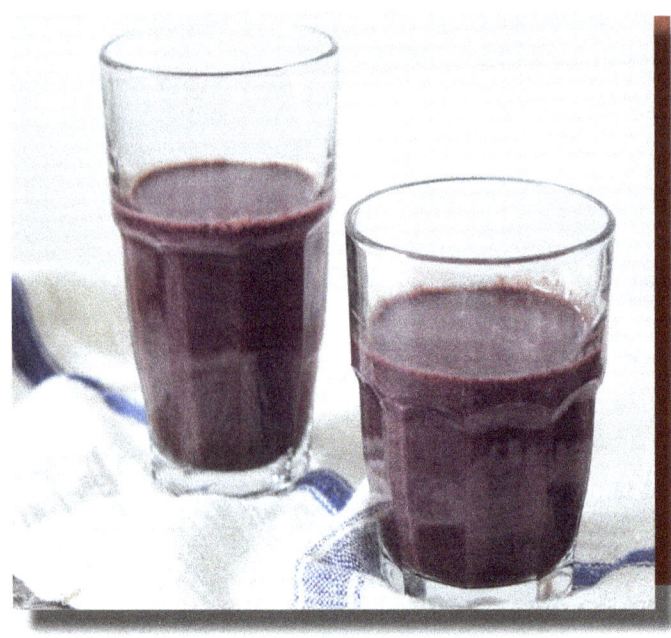

NOTES

In a world filled with processed foods and artificial ingredients, these alkaline recipes offer a refreshing reminder of the power of whole, natural foods to heal and nourish.

INSTRUCTIONS

1. Blend spinach and almond milk first. Then add the remaining ingredients except chia seeds, and blend.

2. Add chia seeds once smooth, then blend on a very low speed to mix. If you don't have a variable-speed blender, mix chia seeds with the rest of the ingredients by hand.

3. Let sit for a few minutes for the chia seeds to expand, then enjoy.

KALE PESTO
PASTA

RECIPE 10

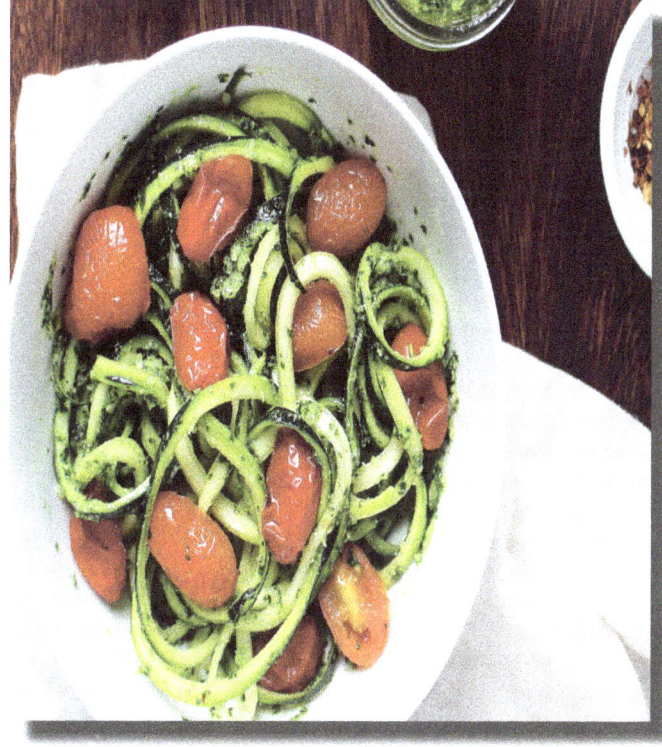

INGREDIENTS

1 bunch Kale

2 cups Fresh Basil

1/4 cup Extra Virgin Olive Oil

1/2 cup Walnuts

2 Limes, fresh squeezed

Sea Salt and Pepper

1 Zucchini, noodled (spiralizer)

Optional: garnish with sliced asparagus

- spinach leaves, and tomato

INSTRUCTIONS

1. The night before, soak walnuts to improve absorption. Put all ingredients in a blender or food processor, and blend until you get a creamy consistency. Add to zucchini noodles and enjoy!

NOTES

Nourish your body with the gentle flow of alkaline water, infusing each sip with love and gratitude. Feel the loving embrace of hydration as it cascades through your cells, replenishing and revitalizing your spirit from within, as you embrace the present moment with tenderness and compassion as you journey into the depths of your own heart and soul. Let each breath be a loving reminder of your inner peace, guiding you towards serenity and inner harmony.

APPLE AND ALMOND BUTTER
OATS

RECIPE 11

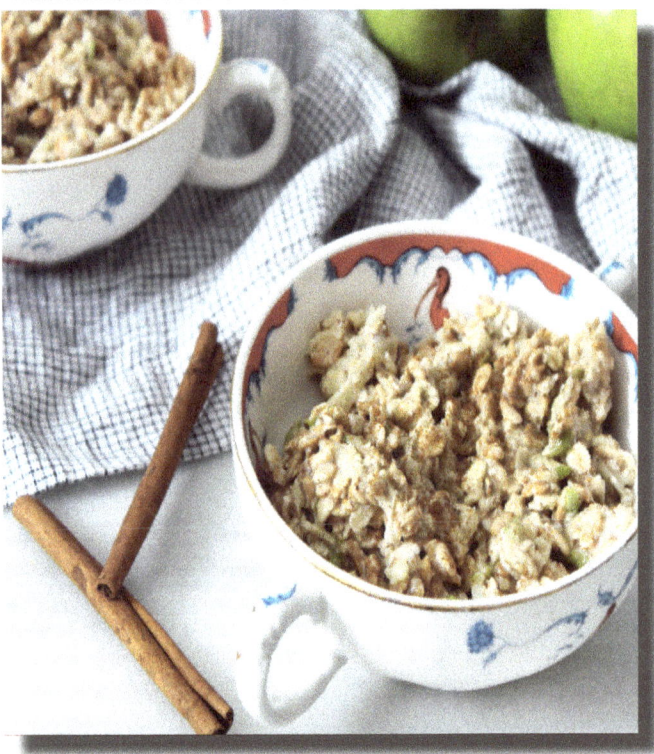

INGREDIENTS

2 cups Gluten-Free Oats

1½ cups Coconut Milk

1/3 cup Raw Almond Butter

1 cup Grated Green Apple

1 tsp Cinnamon Powder

INSTRUCTIONS

1. Mix the oats, coconut milk, and almond butter to a bowl.

2. Stir in the grated apple, cover the bowl with a lid or plastic wrap, and place it in the refrigerator. Refrigerate overnight. If the oats get too thick, add some coconut milk to them.
Garnish with cinnamon powder.

NOTES

Surrender to the loving embrace of sleep, allowing its gentle currents to carry you into the depths of rest and rejuvenation. As you drift into dreams, feel the tender whispers of your soul guiding you toward inner peace and restoration. Loving yourself through all of the phases in life will allow you to truly rest.

GREEN GODDESS BOWL WITH AVOCADO CUMIN **DRESSING**

RECIPE 12

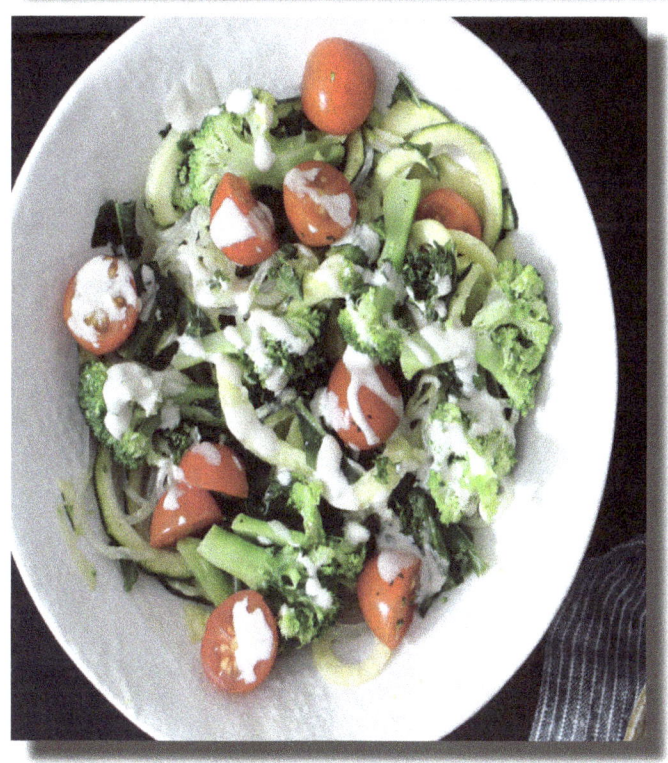

INGREDIENTS

1 Avocado

1 tbsp Cumin Powder

2 Limes, fresh squeezed

1 cup Filtered Water

1/4 tsp Sea Salt

1 tbsp Extra Virgin Olive Oil

Dash Cayenne Pepper

Optional: 1/4 tsp Smoked Paprika

INGREDIENTS FOR TAHINI LEMON DRESSING

-1/4 cup Tahini (sesame butter)

-1/2 cup Filtered Water (less for thicker)

- 3/4 tsp Sea Salt (Celtic grey, :
- Himalayan, Redmond Real Salt)

-1 tbsp Extra Virgin Olive Oil

-Black Pepper to taste

INGREDIENTS FOR SALAD

-3 cups Kale, chopped

-1/2 cup Broccoli Florets, chopped

-1/2 Zucchini noodled (spiralizer)

-1/2 cup Kelp Noodles, soaked and drained

-1/3 cup Cherry Tomatoes, halved

-2 tbsp Hemp Seeds

INSTRUCTIONS

1. Lightly steam kale and broccoli (flash steam for 4 minutes), set aside.

2. Mix zucchini noodles and kelp noodles and toss with a generous serving of avocado cumin dressing.

3. Add cherry tomatoes and toss again. Plate the steamed kale and broccoli and drizzle them with lemon tahini dressing. Top kale and broccoli with the dressed noodles and tomatoes and sprinkle

NOTES

Let these recipes be a celebration of your commitment to self-care and self-love. With each meal, you are affirming your worth and your dedication to living your best life.

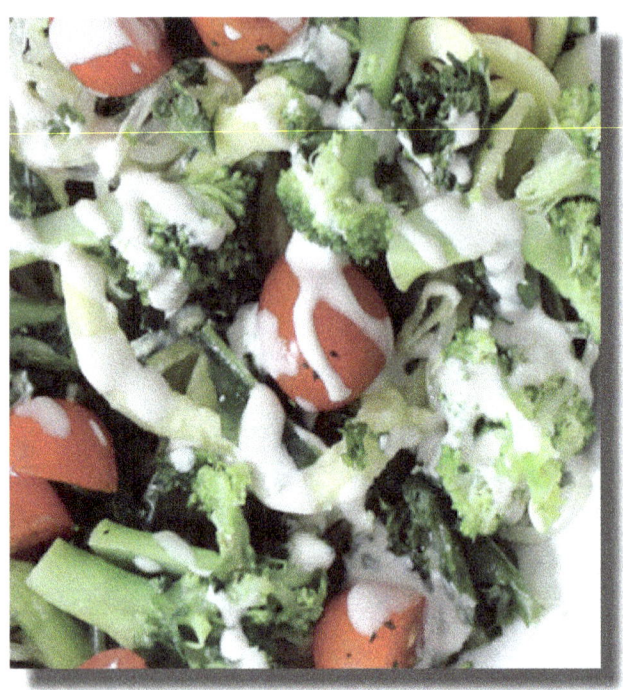

BERRY GOOD SPINACH POWER **SMOOTHIE**

RECIPE 13

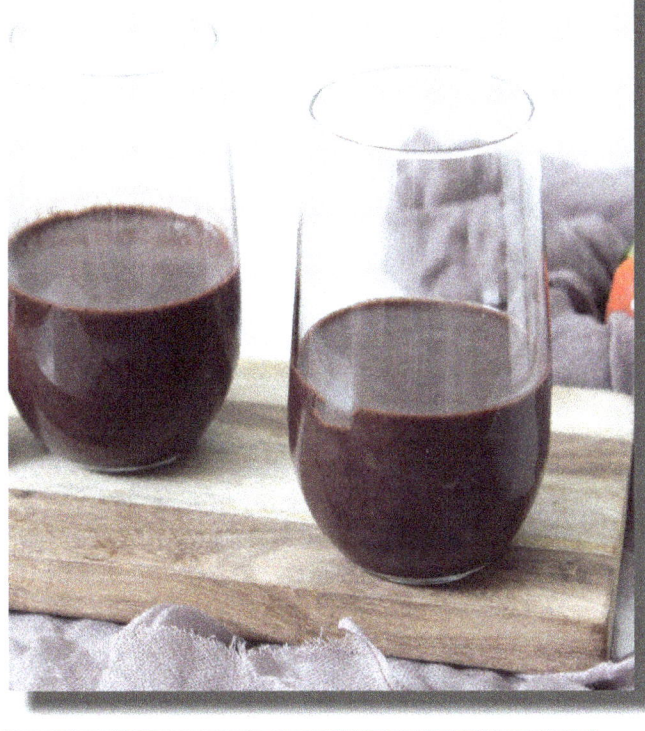

INGREDIENTS

2 cups Fresh Spinach

2 cups Unsweetened Almond Milk

1 cup Frozen Mixed Berries

1 Frozen Banana

1 tbsp Coconut Oil

1/2 tsp Powder

2 tbsp Raw Almond Butter

INSTRUCTIONS

1. Blend spinach and almond milk first, then add the remaining ingredients and blend.

NOTES

There is beauty in simplicity. These alkaline recipes remind us that the most nourishing meals are sometimes made with the fewest ingredients and the purest intentions.

QUINOA BURRITO BOWL

RECIPE 14

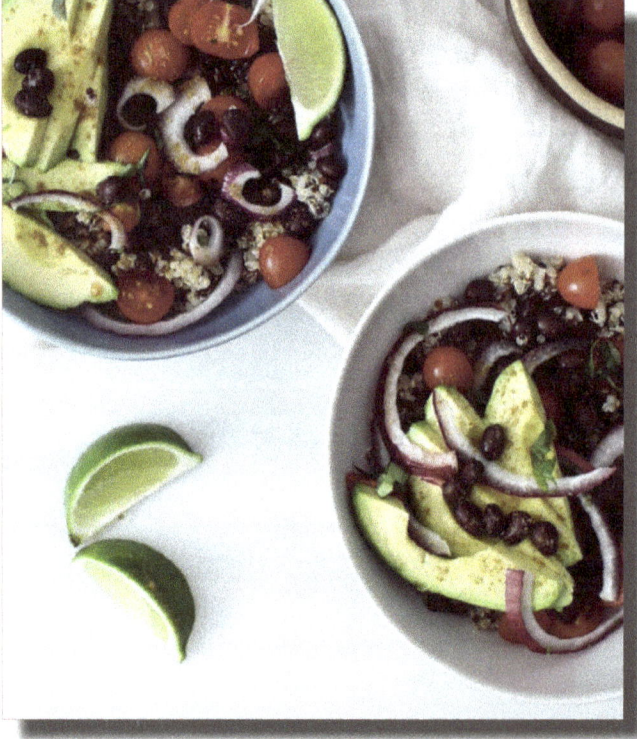

INGREDIENTS

1 cup Quinoa (or brown rice)

2 15-oz cans Black or Adzuki Beans

4 Green Onions (Scallions), sliced

2 Limes, fresh juiced

4 Garlic Cloves, minced

1 heaping tsp. Powder

2 Avocados, sliced

1 small handful of Cilantro, chopped

INSTRUCTIONS

1. Cook quinoa or rice. While cooking, warm beans over low heat.

2. Stir in onions, lime juice, garlic, and cumin, and let flavors combine for 10-15 minutes. When quinoa is done cooking, divide it into one bowl for individual servings. Top with beans, avocado, and cilantro.

NOTES

As you savor these alkaline dishes, please take a moment to pause and express gratitude for the abundance that surrounds you; in gratitude, we find true abundance.

QUINOA MORNING PORRIDGE

RECIPE 15

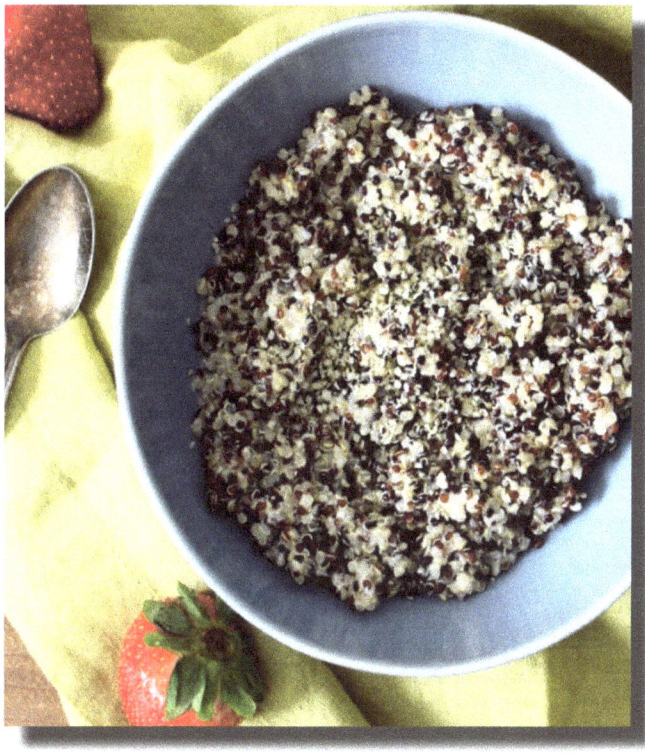

INGREDIENTS

1/2 cup Quinoa, rinsed

1 15 oz can of Coconut Milk

1 tsp Powder

1 tsp Chia Seeds

1 tsp Hemp Seeds

1 heaping tsp. Powder

2 Avocados, sliced

1 small handful of Cilantro, chopped

INSTRUCTIONS

1. Combine all ingredients except hemp seeds and simmer for 10-15 minutes until liquid is absorbed. Sprinkle with hemp seeds.

NOTES

Your body reflects the choices you make each day. Choose health, choose vitality, and choose these alkaline recipes as your allies on the journey to wellness.

THAI QUINOA SALAD

RECIPE 16

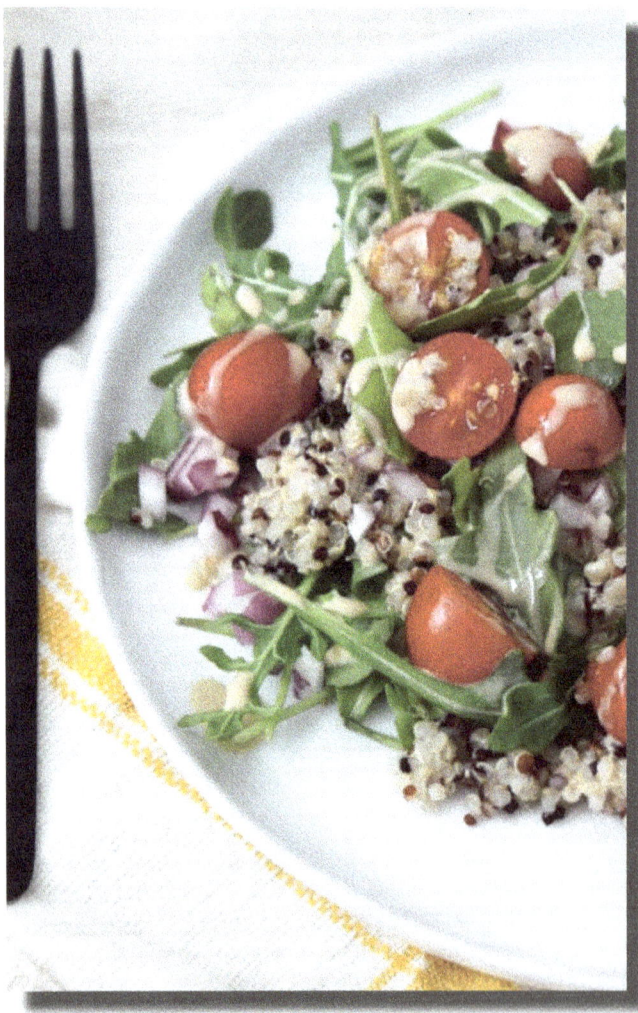

INGREDIENTS

INGREDIENTS FOR DRESSING

- 1 tbsp Sesame Seeds
- 1 tsp Chopped Garlic
- 1 tsp Lemon, fresh juiced
- 3 tsp Apple Cider Vinegar
- 2 tsp Tamari, gluten-free
- 1/4 cup Tahini (sesame butter)
- 1 Date, pitted 1/4 cup shelled Pistachios
- 1/2 tsp Salt
- 1/2 tsp Toasted Sesame Oil

INGREDIENTS FOR SALAD

- 1 cup Quinoa, steamed
- 1 large handful of Arugula
- 1 Tomato, sliced
- 1/4 cup Red Onion, diced

INSTRUCTIONS

1. In a small blender, add the following: ¼ cup + two tbsp filtered water and the rest of the ingredients, and blend.

2. Steam 1 cup of quinoa in a steamer or rice cooker, then set aside.

3. Combine quinoa, arugula, sliced tomatoes, and diced red onion onto a serving plate or bowl.

4. Add Thai dressing, mix by hand with a spoon, and serve.

NOTES

Nourish your body, feed your soul. With each bite of these alkaline-rich recipes, you sow the seeds of vitality and well-being.

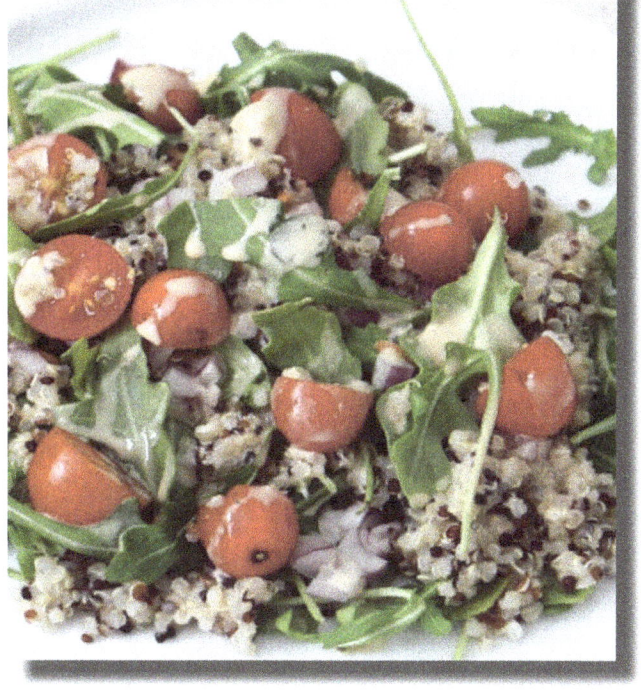

ALKAMIND WARRIOR CHIA
BREAKFAST

RECIPE 17

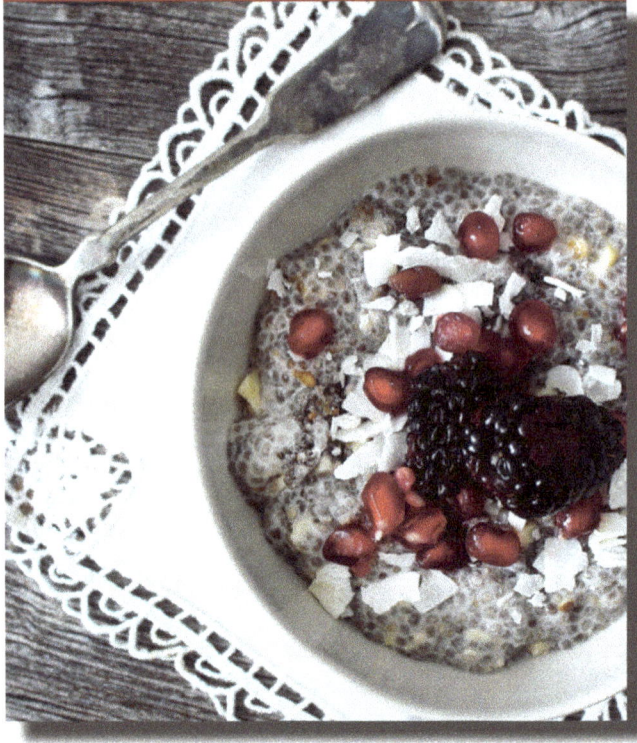

INGREDIENTS

1 cup Unsweetened Almond or Coconut Milk

4 tbsp Chia Seeds

1/2 tsp Vanilla

1/2 tsp Powder

1 tbsp Unsweetened Shredded Coconut Flakes

1/4 cup Chopped Nuts (almonds, cashews or hemp seeds)

INSTRUCTIONS

1. The night before, combine milk and chia seeds in a mason jar. Add vanilla, cinnamon and chopped nuts.

2. Cover with a lid and shake the mixture until combined. Refrigerate overnight. The next morning, shake or stir the mixture and divide it into two or three bowls. Top with optional fresh fruit, coconut shreds, or more chopped nuts.

NOTES

Embrace the healing power of nature's bounty. Let these recipes be a testament to the miracles that can unfold when we honor our bodies with wholesome, alkaline foods.

ASIAN SESAME DRESSING AND **NOODLES**

RECIPE 18

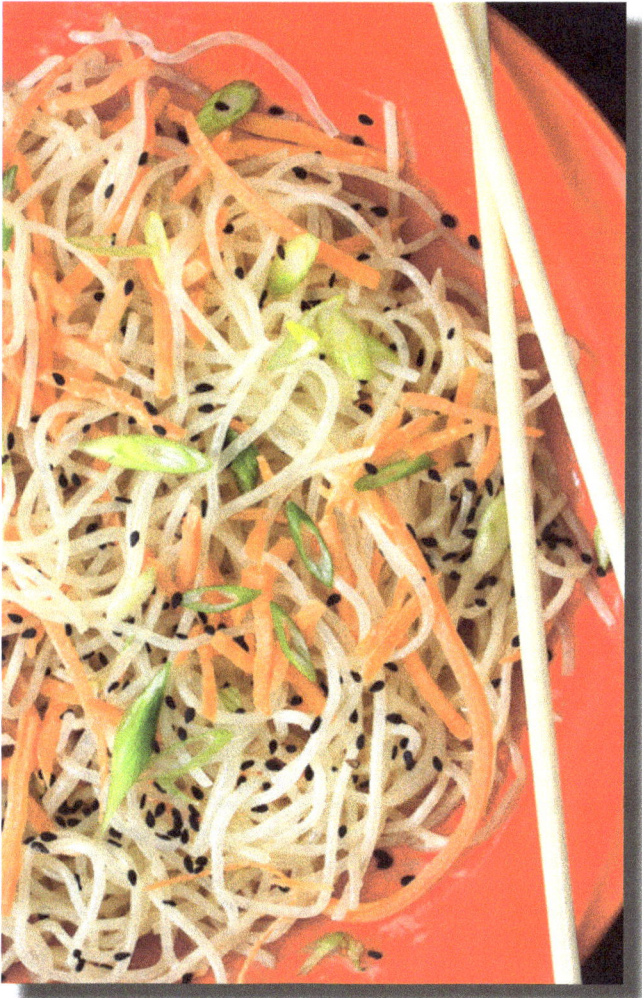

INGREDIENTS

INGREDIENTS FOR DRESSING

- 2 tbsp Tahini (sesame butter)
- 2 tsp Tamari (gluten-free)
- 1/2 tsp Liquid Coconut Nectar (Secrets Brand)
- 3 1/2 tsp Lemon, fresh squeezed 1/4 cup
- 1 Clove Garlic, minced

INGREDIENTS FOR NOODLE SALAD

- 1 Scallion, choppedchopped
- 1 tbsp Raw Sesame Seeds (topping)
- 1/4 cup of each to ingredient
- Optional: 1/4 cup sliced red bell pepper
    - and/or carrot

INSTRUCTIONS

1. Choose one of the following for noodles: Kelp Noodles (1 bag) or 1 Zucchini (use spiralizer or vegetable peeler)

2. In a mixing bowl, combine all the dressing ingredients and thoroughly mix with a spoon.

3. Make your zucchini noodles with a spiralizer or, if using kelp noodles, place in warm water for 10 minutes to rinse off the liquid they are packaged with, allowing them to separate and soften.

4. Add 1/4 cup of thin sliced red bell pepper and 1/4 cup of diced carrots.

5. Add the Asian Sesame dressing to the noodles and scallions, and mix thoroughly. Add sesame seeds on top, and serve.

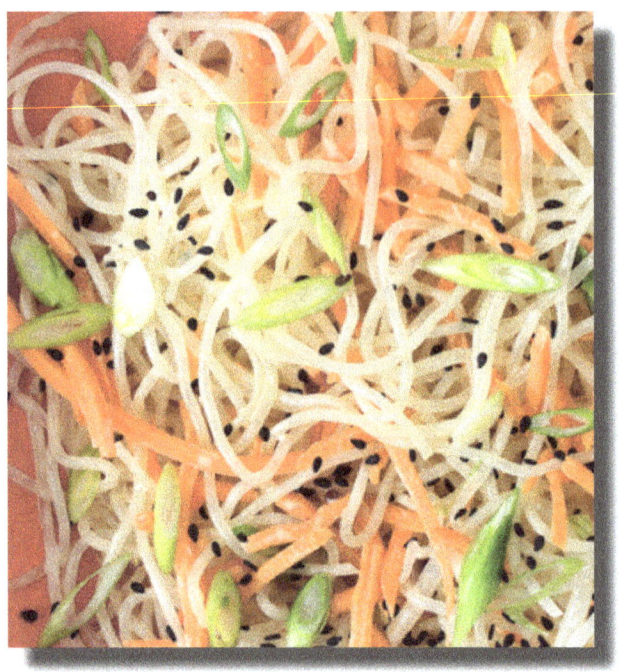

NOTES

In the kitchen, as in life, balance is key. May these recipes serve as a reminder to cultivate balance in all aspects of your being—body, mind, and spirit.

FRENCH TOAST

RECIPE 19

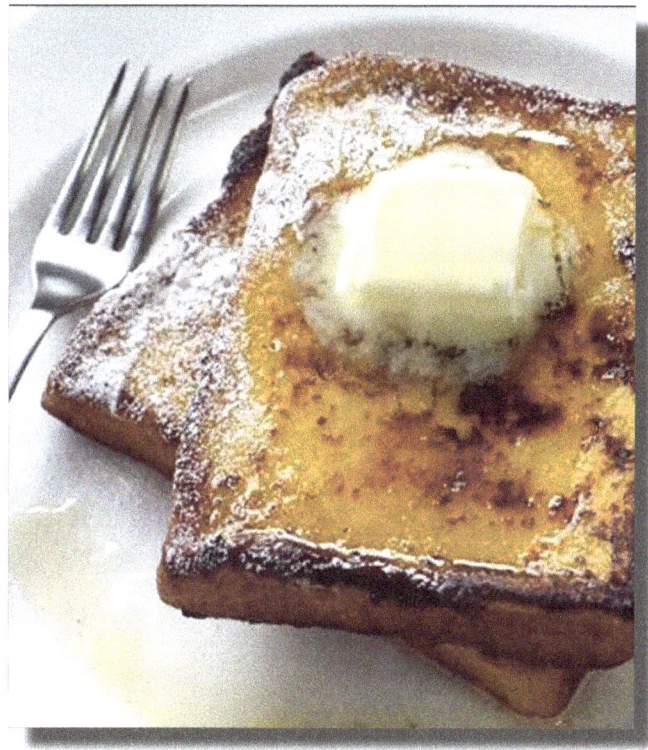

INGREDIENTS

1/2 cup of flour

6 slices of Brown Bread

2 Eggs

1/2 cup of Milk

1 tbs of Ground Cinnamon

1 tsp of Salt for taste

1 tsp of Vanilla

1/4 tsp of Powder

INSTRUCTIONS

1. Beat the eggs, milk, salt, spices, and vanilla in a bowl.

2. Dip the bread in the egg mixture and allow it to soak both sides.

3. Pour some oil into a pan and heat it on low.

4. Cook both sides of the bread until they turn golden.

5. Serve hot with a dollop of butter.

NOTES

Find a place near you to hold space for the soothing warmth of sauna sessions. These sessions allow your body to gently release toxins through a loving sweat. Feel the tension melt away as you envelop yourself in nurturing heat, promoting relaxation and renewal as you continue to nourish yourself from the inside out.

ALKALINE APPLE
PANCAKES

RECIPE 20

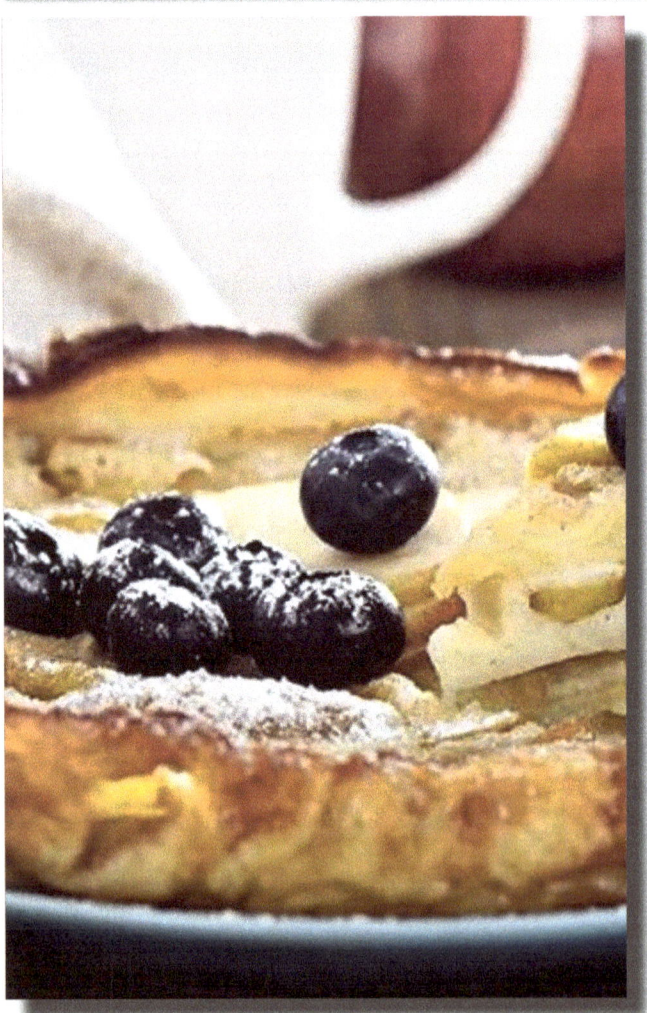

INGREDIENTS

1 cup almond flour

1/4 cup coconut flour

1 teaspoon baking powder

1/2 teaspoon cinnamon

Pinch of sea salt

1 tablespoon maple syrup (optional)

1 teaspoon vanilla extract

1 large apple, grated

Coconut oil for cooking

2 tablespoons ground flaxseed mixed with :

    -6 tablespoons water (flaxseed "egg")

1 cup unsweetened almond milk

INSTRUCTIONS

1. Prepare Flaxseed "Egg": Mix the ground flaxseed and water in a small bowl. Let it sit for 5-10 minutes until it thickens and forms a gel-like consistency.

2, Prepare Dry Ingredients: In a large mixing bowl, whisk together the almond flour, coconut flour, baking powder, cinnamon, and a pinch of sea salt.

3. Combine Wet Ingredients: In another bowl, whisk together the flaxseed "egg," almond milk, maple syrup (if using), and vanilla extract.

4.Grate Apple: Peel and grate the apple using a box grater or a food processor. Squeeze out any excess liquid from the grated apple using a clean kitchen towel or paper towel.

5. Mix Batter: Add the grated apple to the wet ingredients and mix well. Then, pour the wet ingredients into the bowl with the dry ingredients. Stir until just combined, being careful not to over-mix.

6. Cook Pancakes: Heat a non-stick skillet or griddle over medium heat and lightly grease with coconut oil. Once the skillet is hot, pour about 1/4 cup of batter onto the skillet for each pancake. Use the back of a spoon to spread the batter into a circle.

7. Cook until Bubbles Form: Cook the pancakes for 2-3 minutes or until bubbles form on the surface and the edges start to look set.

8. Flip and Cook: Carefully flip the pancakes using a spatula and cook for an additional 1-2 minutes on the other side or until golden brown and cooked through.

9. Serve: Transfer the cooked pancakes to a plate and repeat with the remaining batter. Serve the pancakes warm with your favorite toppings, such as sliced bananas, berries, chopped nuts, or a drizzle of maple syrup.

NOTES

Practice active listening in your interactions with others today. Love. Focus entirely on the person speaking without interrupting or formulating a response in your mind. Notice the tone of their voice, their body language, and the emotions behind their words. Mindful listening can deepen your connections with others and foster empathy.

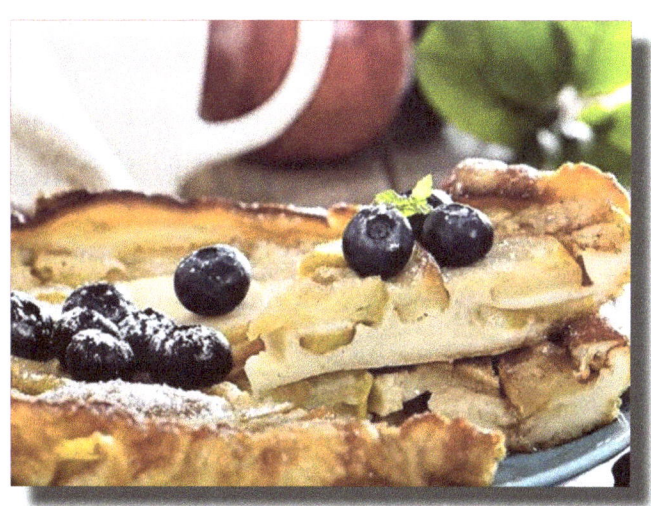

ALKALINE
TORTILLAS

RECIPE 21

INGREDIENTS

2 cups almond flour

1/4 cup arrowroot powder

1/4 teaspoon sea salt

2 tablespoons olive oil

Warm water, as needed

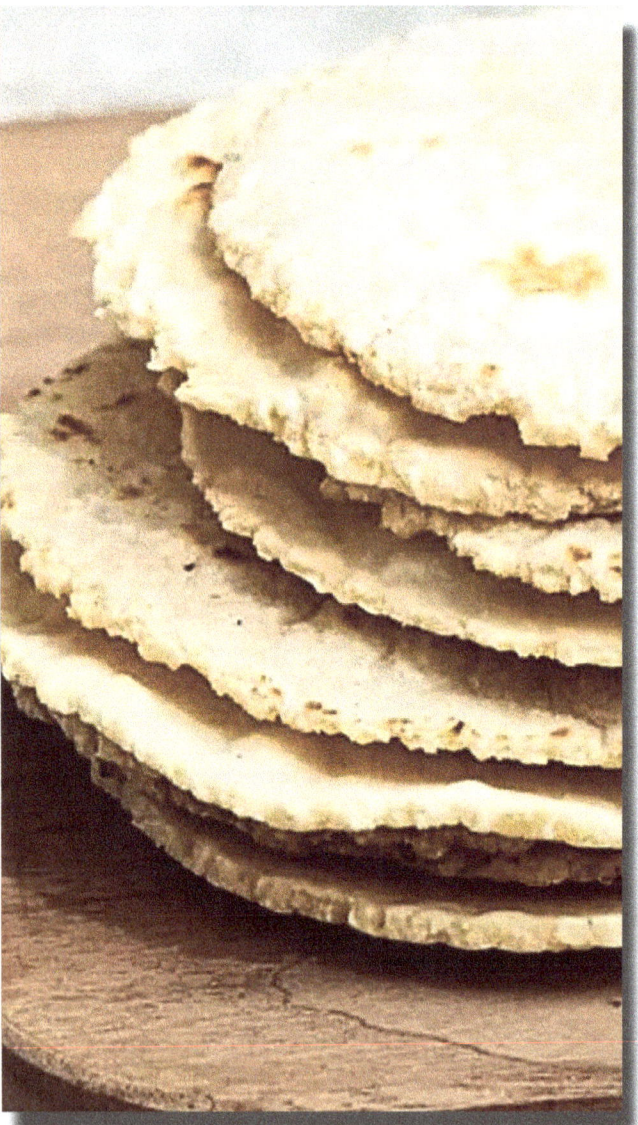

INSTRUCTIONS

1. Mix Dry Ingredients: In a mixing bowl, combine the almond flour, arrowroot powder, and sea salt. Stir until well combined.

2, Add Olive Oil: Drizzle the olive oil over the dry ingredients and mix until the mixture resembles coarse crumbs.

3. Add Water: Gradually add warm water, a little at a time, while stirring the mixture with a spoon or your hands. Add water until a dough forms and holds together without being too sticky or dry.

4. Knead Dough: Transfer the dough onto a clean surface and knead it for a few minutes until it becomes smooth and elastic.

5. Divide Dough: Divide the dough into eight equal portions and shape each portion into a ball.

6. Roll Out Tortillas: Place a dough ball between two sheets of parchment paper or plastic wrap. Use a rolling pin to flatten the dough into a thin, round tortilla, about 6-8 inches in diameter. Repeat with the remaining dough balls.

7. Cook Tortillas: Heat a non-stick skillet or griddle over medium heat. Once hot, carefully transfer a tortilla onto the skillet and cook for about 1-2 minutes on each side or until lightly golden brown spots appear. Repeat with the remaining tortillas.

8. Serve: Serve the tortillas warm with your favorite toppings or fillings, such as grilled vegetables, beans, avocado, salsa, or hummus.

9. These alkaline tortillas are versatile. They can be used to make wraps, tacos, and quesadillas or enjoyed independently. Experiment with different fillings and flavors to create delicious and nutritious meals.

NOTES

Take time to savor each bite of your meals. Notice the food's colors, textures, and flavors on your plate. Chew slowly and pay attention to the sensations of taste and smell as you eat. Eating mindfully can enhance your enjoyment of food and promote better digestion.

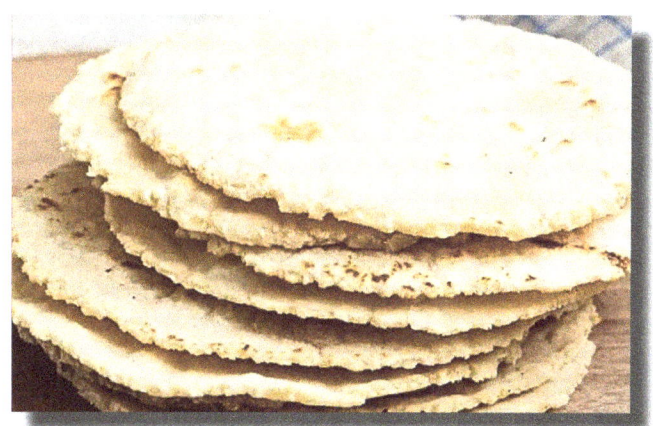

ALKALINE AVOCADO BREAKFAST **TOAST**

RECIPE 22

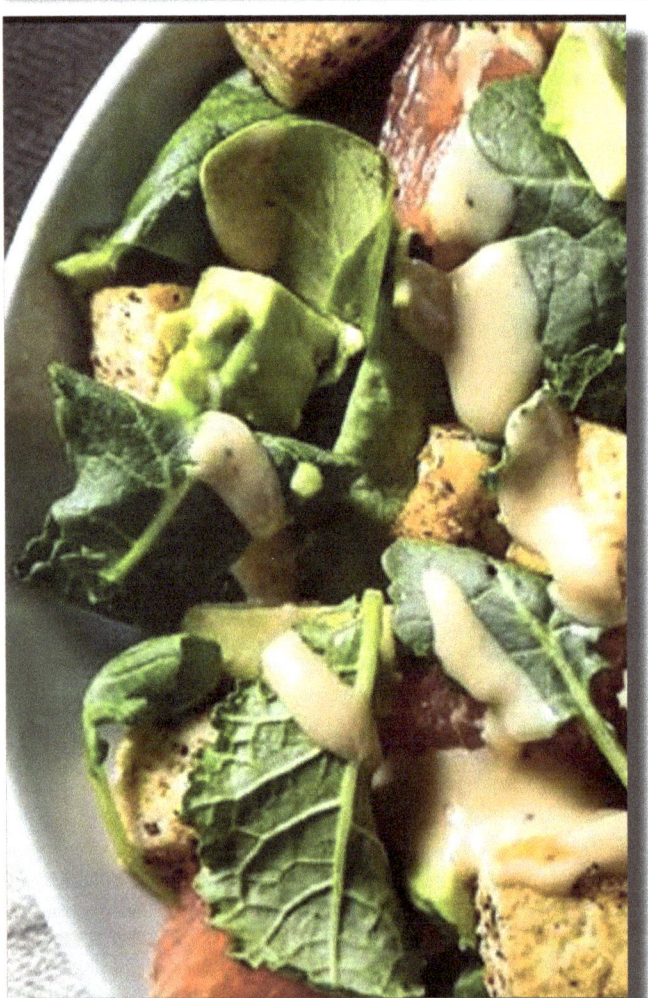

INGREDIENTS

1 ripe avocado

1 small tomato, sliced

Handful of alfalfa sprouts or micro greens

Lemon juice

Sea salt and black pepper to taste

2 slices of alkaline bread:
- (such as spelt bread or sprouted grain bread)

Optional toppings: sliced radishes,
- hemp seeds, nutritional yeast, or chili flakes

INSTRUCTIONS

1. Prepare Avocado: Cut the ripe avocado in half and remove the pit. Scoop the avocado flesh into a small bowl.

2, Mash Avocado: Mash it with a fork until smooth, or leave it slightly chunky if desired.

3.Toast Bread: Toast the slices of alkaline bread until golden brown and crispy.

ASSEMBLE TOAST

- Spread the mashed avocado evenly onto the toasted bread slices.

- Arrange the sliced tomato on top of the avocado spread.

- Sprinkle with a squeeze of lemon juice, sea salt, and black pepper to taste.

- Add Toppings: Garnish the avocado toast with a handful of alfalfa sprouts or microgreens for extra freshness and crunch.

- Optional Toppings: For added flavor and nutrition, you can sprinkle your avocado toast with sliced radishes, hemp seeds, nutritional yeast, or chili flakes.

- Serve: Serve the avocado breakfast toast immediately while the bread is warm and crisp.

NOTES

1. Enjoy the distinct mixture and potency of an incredible yet simplistic combination. Much like life, there is a reward in finding the seemingly simple wonders of the day.

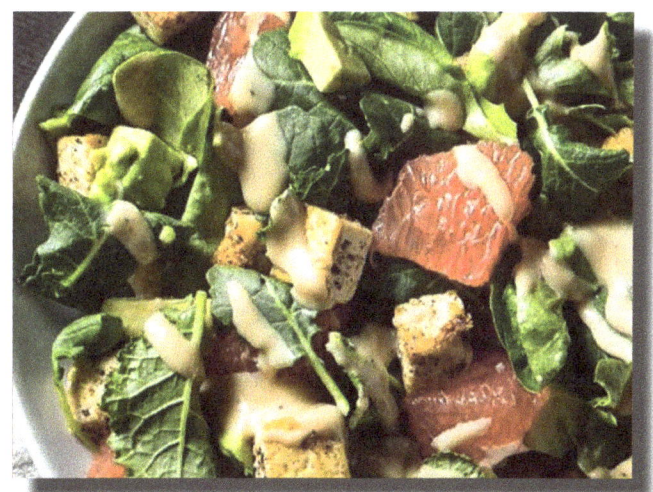

LATIN AMERICAN STYLE ALKALINE MIXED SPROUT SALAD WITH ALKALINE TORTILLAS

RECIPE 23

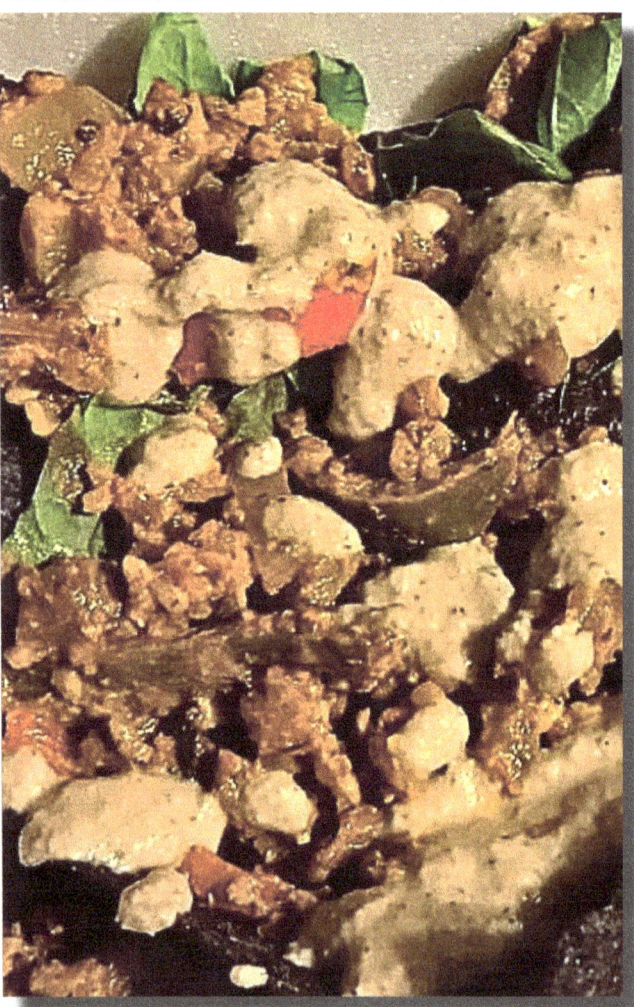

INGREDIENTS

For the Salad:

- 2 cups mixed sprouts (such as mung bean sprouts, lentil sprouts, and chickpea sprouts)
- 1 cup cherry tomatoes, halved
- 1 bell pepper, diced
- 1/2 red onion, thinly sliced
- 1 avocado, diced
- 1/4 cup cilantro, chopped
- Juice of 1 lime
- Salt and pepper to taste

For the Dressing:
- 2 tablespoons olive oil
- 1 tablespoon apple cider vinegar
- 1 teaspoon maple syrup (optional)
- 1 teaspoon ground cumin
- 1/2 teaspoon smoked paprika
- Salt and pepper to taste

Alkaline tortillas (prepared using the previous recipe)
Lime wedges
Extra cilantro for garnish

INSTRUCTIONS

1. Prepare the Salad: In a large mixing bowl, combine the mixed sprouts, cherry tomatoes, bell pepper, red onion, avocado, and cilantro.

2. Make the Dressing: In a small bowl, whisk together the olive oil, apple cider vinegar, maple syrup (if using), ground cumin, smoked paprika, salt, and pepper until well combined.

3. Combine Salad and Dressing: Pour the dressing over the salad ingredients in the mixing bowl. Toss gently until everything is evenly coated with the dressing. Adjust seasoning with salt and pepper if needed.

Assemble Alkaline Tortillas:

- Warm the prepared alkaline tortillas in a skillet or microwave until heated through. Place them on a serving platter.

- Serve: Serve the mixed sprout salad alongside the warm, alkaline tortillas. Garnish with extra cilantro and lime wedges for squeezing over the salad and tortillas.

- Enjoy: To enjoy, scoop some of the mixed sprout salad onto an alkaline tortilla, fold it over like a taco or wrap, and take a bite! The freshness of the sprouts, combined with the tangy dressing and soft tortillas, creates a delicious and nutritious meal inspired by Latin American flavors.

NOTES

This Latin American-style alkaline mixed sprout salad is delicious and packed with nutrients and alkaline-forming ingredients. Enjoy it as a light and refreshing meal for lunch or dinner!

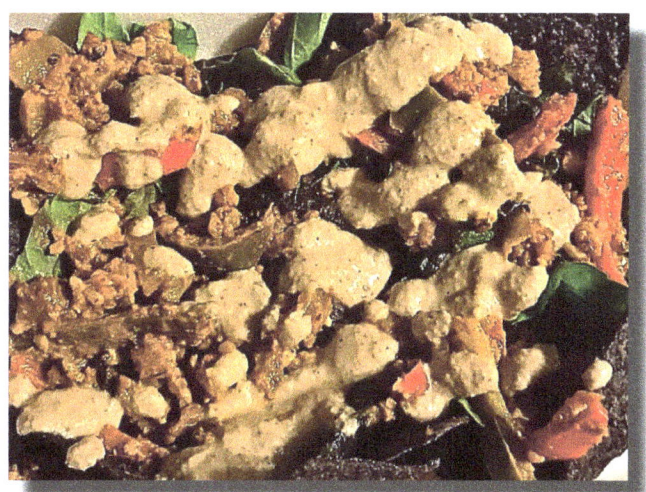

ALKALINE KALE AND CHICKPEA HUMMUS

RECIPE 24

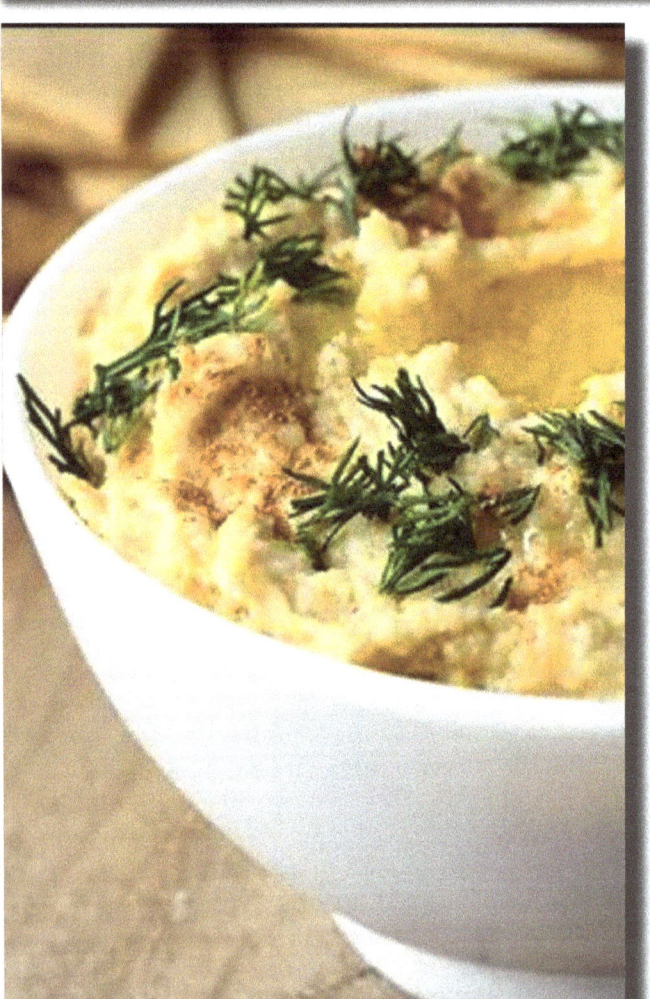

INGREDIENTS

1 bunch kale, stems removed: - and leaves chopped

1 can (15 oz) chickpeas, rinsed and drained

2 cloves garlic, minced

2 tablespoons extra virgin olive oil

Juice of 1 lemon

Salt and pepper to taste

-Juice of 1 lime

-Salt and pepper to taste

Optional: red pepper flakes or paprika for added flavor

Alkaline tortillas (prepared using the previous recipe)
Lime wedges
Extra cilantro for garnish

INSTRUCTIONS

1. Prepare Kale: Bring a large pot of salted water to a boil. Add the chopped kale leaves to the boiling water and cook for 3-5 minutes or until tender. Drain the kale and set aside.

2. Cook Chickpeas: Heat one tablespoon of olive oil over medium heat in a small saucepan. Add the minced garlic and cook for 1-2 minutes or until fragrant. Add the rinsed and drained chickpeas to the saucepan and cook for 5-7 minutes, stirring occasionally, until heated and slightly crispy.

3. Mash Ingredients: Combine the cooked kale and chickpeas in a large mixing bowl. Mash the mixture with a potato masher or fork until it reaches your desired consistency. You can leave it slightly chunky or mash it until smooth.

4. Season: Drizzle the remaining one tablespoon of olive oil over the mashed kale and chickpeas. Squeeze the lemon juice over the mixture and season with salt, pepper, and any optional spices such as red pepper flakes or paprika. Stir well to combine and adjust the seasoning to taste.

5. Serve: Transfer the mashed kale and chickpeas to a serving dish. Enjoy it warm as a side dish, or spread it on toast for a hearty and nutritious breakfast or snack.

6. Optional Garnish: Before serving, garnish the mashed kale and chickpeas with a drizzle of extra virgin olive oil and a sprinkle of fresh herbs like parsley or cilantro.

NOTES

This alkaline kale and chickpea mash is a delicious and nutritious way to enjoy the flavors of kale and chickpeas together. It's packed with fiber, vitamins, and minerals, making it a satisfying and alkaline-friendly dish.

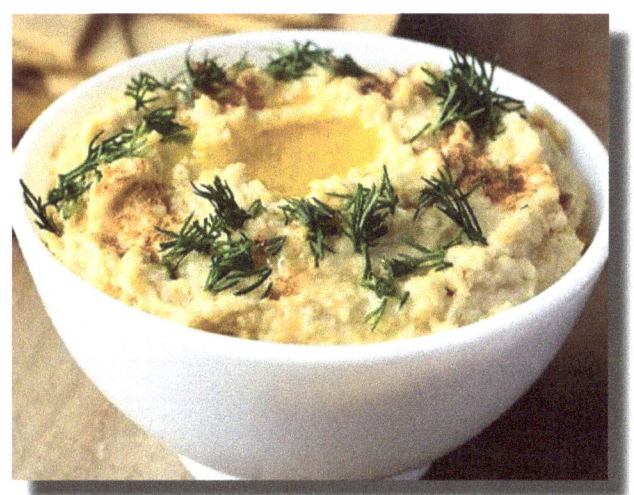

QUINOA AND APPLE
BREAKFAST

RECIPE 25

INGREDIENTS

1/2 cup Quinoa

1 Apple

1/2 Lemon

1 pinch Powder

NOTES

You deserve a magical life and are getting closer to it with every alkaline bite you take.

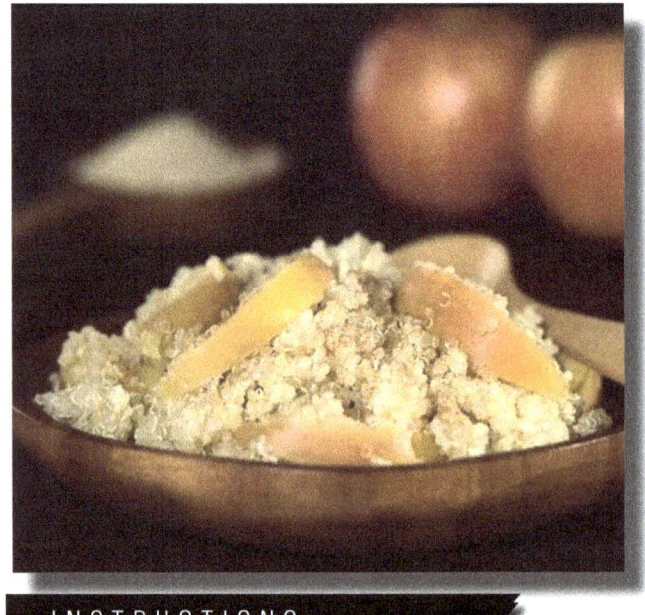

INSTRUCTIONS

1. Cook the quinoa according to the instructions on the packet.

2. Add some water. Boil and simmer for 15 minutes.

3. Grate the apple, add it to the quinoa, and cook for another 30 seconds.

4. IServe in a bowl. Sprinkle cinnamon on top. You can also add raisins.

EASY ALKALINE
YOGURT

RECIPE 26

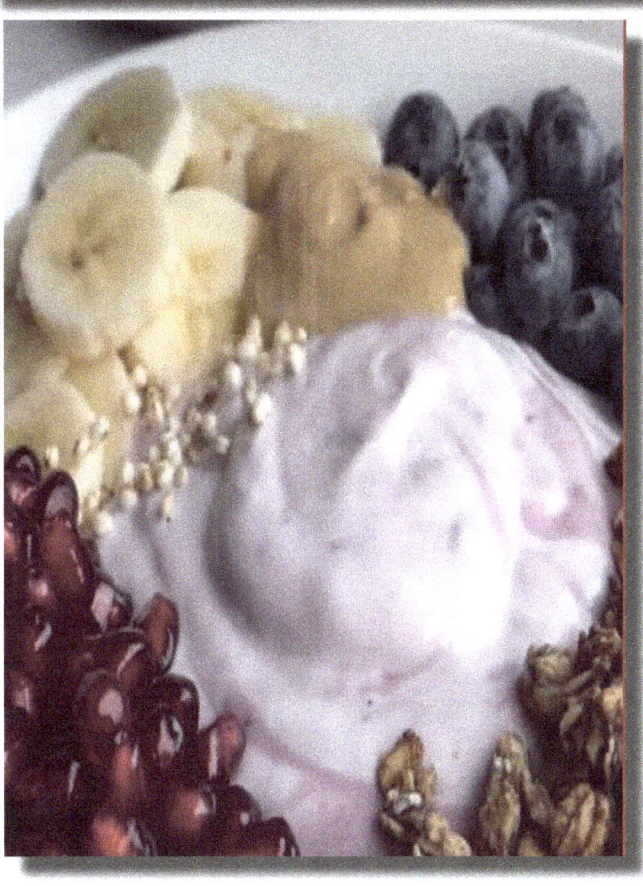

INGREDIENTS

2 cups of unsweetened almond milk or coconut milk

1 tablespoon of agar agar powder (a plant-based gelatin substitute will work)

2-3 tablespoons of lemon juice

1-2 tablespoons of agave syrup (optional for sweetness)

Probiotic capsules or powder (containing Lactobacillus acidophilus or Bifidobacterium lactis strains)

INSTRUCTIONS

1. Prepare the Milk: In a saucepan, heat the almond milk or coconut milk over medium heat until it simmers, being careful not to boil it.

2, Add Agar Agar: Once the milk is simmering, sprinkle the agar agar powder evenly over the surface of the milk. Whisk continuously to dissolve the agar agar powder into the milk. Let it simmer for 2-3 minutes, stirring frequently, until the mixture thickens slightly.

3. Cool the Mixture: Remove the saucepan from the heat and let the mixture cool to around 110°F (43°C). This temperature is important for activating the probiotics later.

4. Add Lemon Juice and Sweetener: Stir in the lemon juice and maple syrup or agave syrup (if using) into the cooled milk mixture. The lemon juice adds a tangy flavor and helps to activate the fermentation process.

5. Add Probiotics: Open the probiotic capsules or measure the probiotic powder and sprinkle it over the milk mixture. Use a clean utensil to stir the probiotics into the mixture gently.

6. Fermentation: Pour the milk mixture into a clean glass jar or container. Cover the jar with a clean kitchen towel or cheesecloth, securing it with a rubber band. Place the jar in a warm spot, such as on top of the refrigerator or in an oven with the light on, and let it ferment for 12-24 hours. The longer it ferments, the tangier and thicker the yogurt will become.

7. Chill and Serve: Once the yogurt has fermented to your desired taste and consistency, transfer it to the refrigerator for at least 2 hours before serving. It will continue to thicken as it chills.

8. Enjoy: You can serve your homemade alkaline yogurt plain or with your favorite toppings, such as fresh fruit, nuts, seeds, or a drizzle of honey or maple syrup.

9. This easy homemade alkaline yogurt is rich in probiotics and free from dairy and added sugars, making it a healthy and delicious addition to your alkaline diet!

NOTES

In your daily life, set aside time each day to write in a journal. Use this time to reflect on your thoughts, feelings, and experiences without judgment. Write down anything that comes to mind, whether it's worries, goals, or moments of joy. Journaling can help you gain insight into your inner world and promote self-awareness.

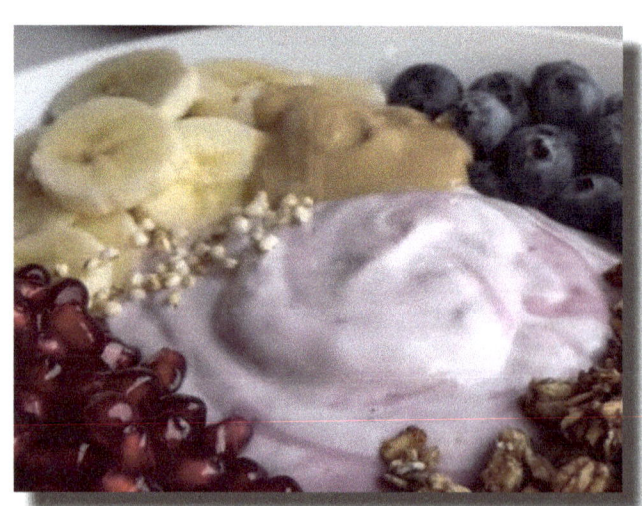

YUMMY COLD OATS

RECIPE 27

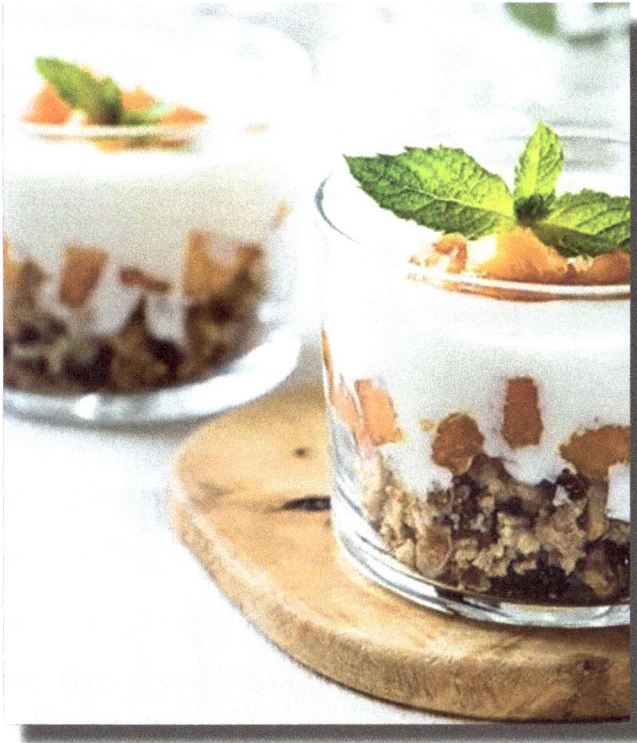

INGREDIENTS

1/2 cup Oats

1/2 cup almond or walnut milk

1/2 cup alkaline yogurt

1/2 tsp Powder

1/2 Banana, sliced

1/2 tbsp Peanut Butter

1/2 cup Berries

INSTRUCTIONS

1. The night before, combine milk and chia seeds in a mason jar. Add vanilla, cinnamon and chopped nuts.

2. Cover with lid and shake the mixture until combined. Refrigerate overnight. The next morning, shake or stir the mixture and divide into 2 or 3 bowls. Top with optional fresh fruit, coconut shreds or more chopped nuts.

NOTES

Embrace the healing power of nature's bounty. Let these recipes be a testament to the miracles that can unfold when we honor our bodies with wholesome, alkaline foods.

ALKALINE SCRAMBLED "EGGS" (TOFU SCRAMBLE)

RECIPE 28

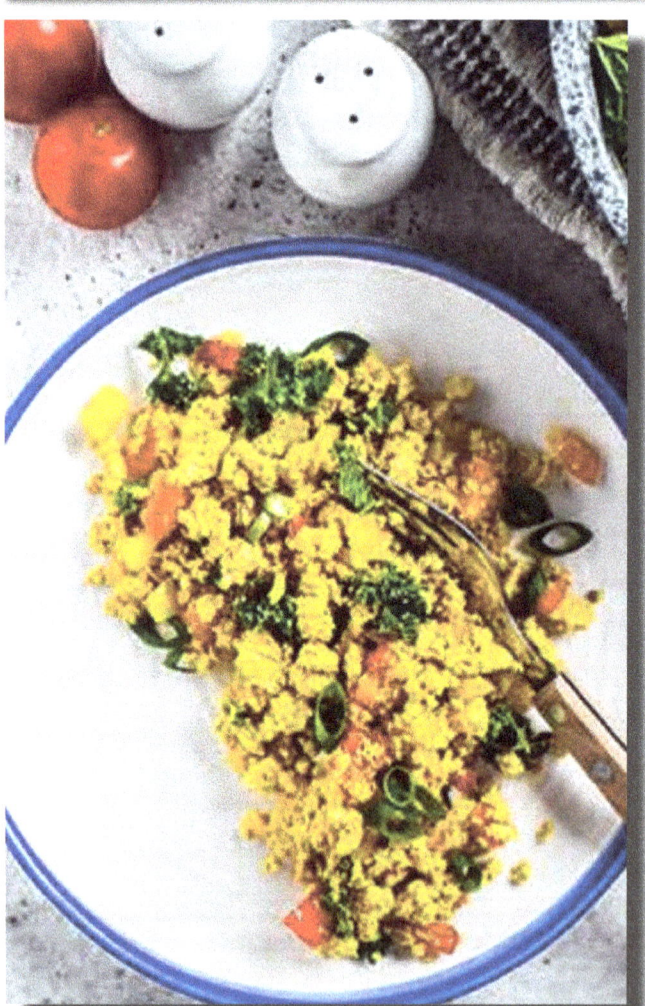

INGREDIENTS

1 block (about 14 oz) of firm tofumilk

1 tablespoon of olive oil or coconut oil

1/4 cup of chopped onion

1/4 cup of chopped bell pepper (any color)

1/4 cup of chopped mushrooms (optional)

1/4 cup of chopped mushrooms (optional)

2 cloves of garlic, minced

1 teaspoon of ground turmeric

1/2 teaspoon of ground cumin

Salt and pepper to taste

Fresh herbs (such as parsley or chives) for garnish

INSTRUCTIONS

1. Prepare Tofu(not alkaline but can be filling): Drain the tofu and pat it dry with paper towels to remove excess moisture. Crumble the tofu into small pieces with your hands or a fork, resembling scrambled eggs.

2, Sauté Vegetables: Heat olive or coconut oil in a skillet over medium heat. Add the chopped onion, bell pepper, and mushrooms (if using) to the skillet. Sauté for 5-7 minutes or until the vegetables are softened.
Add Tofu: Add the crumbled tofu and minced garlic to the skillet with the sautéed vegetables. Stir well to combine.

3. Season: Sprinkle the ground turmeric and ground cumin over the tofu mixture. Stir until the tofu is evenly coated with the spices. The turmeric will color the tofu yellow, similar to scrambled eggs.

4. Cook: Continue to cook the tofu mixture for 5-7 minutes, stirring occasionally, until the tofu is heated through and slightly browned.

5. Season to Taste: Season the scrambled "eggs" with salt and pepper to taste. Adjust the seasoning as needed.

6. Garnish: Remove the skillet from the heat. Sprinkle fresh herbs, such as parsley or chives, over the scrambled "eggs" for garnish.

7. Serve: Serve the hot alkaline scrambled "eggs" with your favorite alkaline-friendly sides, such as sliced avocado, steamed greens, or whole-grain toast.

NOTES

This alkaline scrambled tofu is a nutritious and delicious alternative to traditional scrambled eggs, packed with protein and flavor. Enjoy it as a satisfying breakfast or brunch option as part of your alkaline diet!

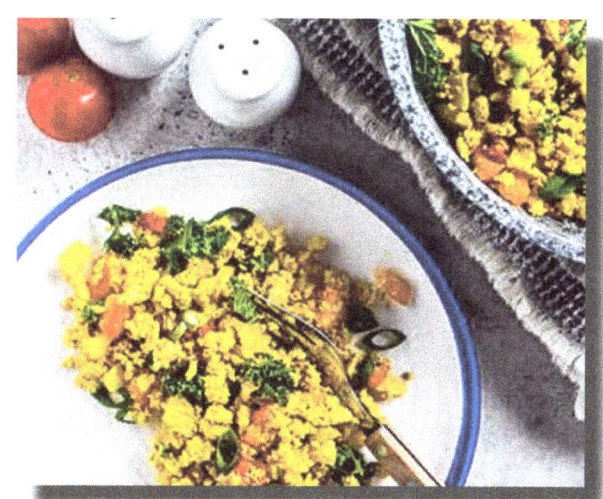

THEPLAS WITH AN ALKALINE TWIST

RECIPE 29

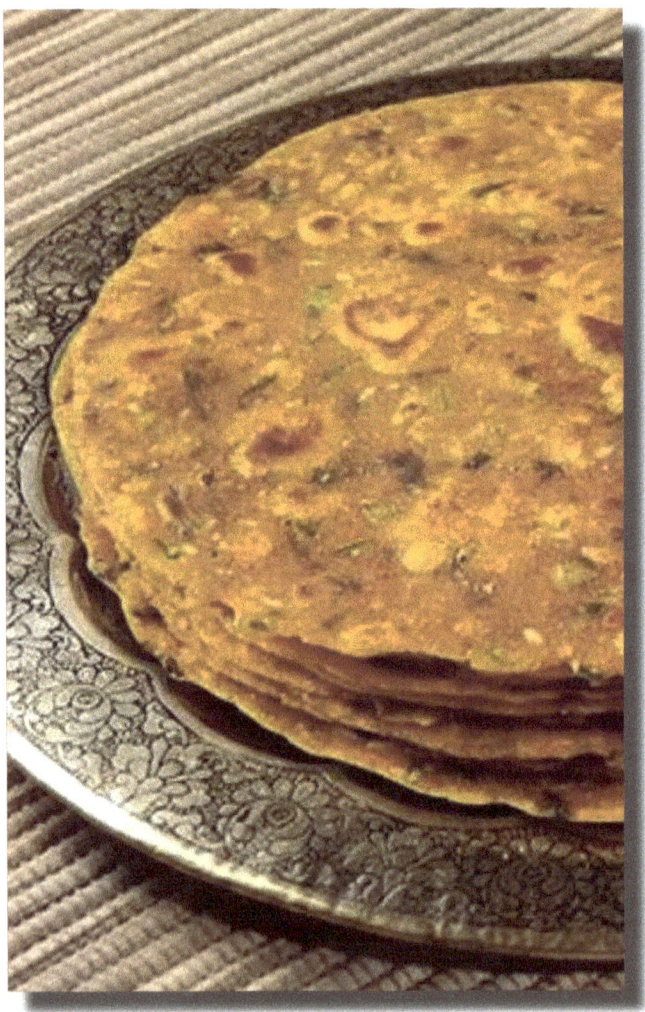

INGREDIENTS

1 cup chickpea flour (besan)

1 cup amaranth flour

1/2 cup chopped spinach leaves

1/4 cup chopped cilantro (coriander) leaves

1/4 cup grated zucchini

2 tablespoons grated ginger

1 green chili, finely chopped (optional)

1 teaspoon ground cumin

1/2 teaspoon ground turmeric

1/2 teaspoon ground coriander

1/4 teaspoon asafoetida (hing)

Salt to taste

1 tablespoon olive oil or coconut oil

Warm water, as needed

Extra flour for rolling

INSTRUCTIONS

1. Prepare Dough: In a large mixing bowl, combine the chickpea flour, amaranth flour, chopped spinach, chopped cilantro, grated zucchini, grated ginger, chopped green chili (if using), ground cumin, ground turmeric, ground coriander, asafoetida, salt, and olive oil. Mix well to combine all the ingredients.

2, Knead Dough: Gradually add warm water to the flour mixture, a little at a time, and knead to form a soft and smooth dough. The dough should be firm but pliable. Add more water or flour as needed to achieve the right consistency.

3. Rest Dough: Cover the dough with a clean kitchen towel or plastic wrap and let it rest for about 15-20 minutes. This allows the dough to relax and makes it easier to roll out.

4. Divide Dough: After resting, divide the dough into small lemon-sized balls. Roll each ball between your palms to make them smooth.

5. Roll Out Theplas: Take one dough ball and flatten it slightly with your palms. Dust it with some flour and roll it into a thin, round thepla using a rolling pin. Repeat with the remaining dough balls.

6. Cook Theplas: Heat a non-stick skillet or griddle over medium heat. Place a rolled-out thepla onto the hot skillet and cook for about 1-2 minutes on each side or until golden brown spots appear and thepla is cooked through. Brush olive or coconut oil on both sides while cooking, if desired.

7. Serve: Serve the hot alkaline theplas with a twist with your favorite alkaline-friendly side dish or condiment, such as yogurt, chutney, or pickle.

8. These alkaline theplas with a twist are nutritious, flavorful, and versatile. They make a delicious breakfast, snack, or light meal option for your alkaline diet!

9. With each recipe you prepare, may you be reminded of your boundless potential and the infinite possibilities that lie ahead. You are a radiant being, capable of achieving anything you set your mind to.

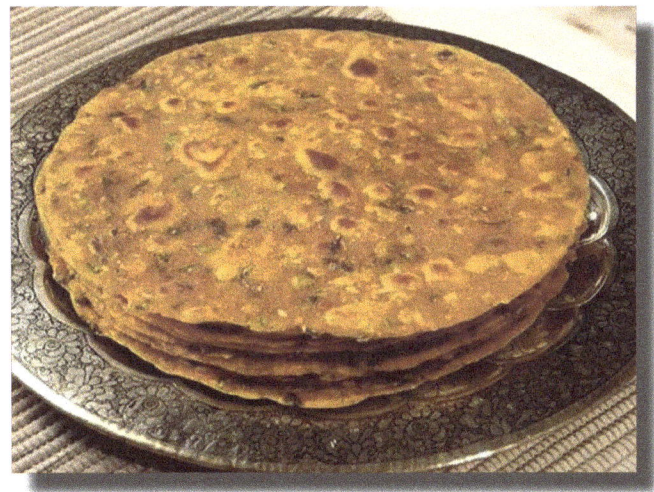

INSTRUCTIONS II

A Few Quick Snacks

- Stir-fry! alkaline vegetables such as broccoli, bell peppers, mushrooms, and snap peas or (or any other) in coconut oil with garlic and ginger. Serve over quinoa for a quick 15-minute meal. With fresh pressed juice!

- Veggie Wraps! Using our Tortilla recipe, Fill the tortilla with hummus, mixed greens, shredded carrots, cucumber slices, avocado, and sprouts for a quick and easy, delicious meal that won't weigh you down and can be eaten on the go.

- Zucchini Pasta! Spiralize zucchini into noodles and toss with alkaline pesto made from basil, pine nuts, garlic, olive oil, and salt to taste. Top with cherry tomatoes and olives for extra flavor. It takes 10 minutes, and you will have no regrets. It is fun to make.

- Quinoa and Alkaline Veggies! Cook quinoa according to package instructions and mix it with chopped vegetables like bell peppers, mushrooms, tomatoes, cucumbers, and avocado. Drizzle with olive oil, lemon juice, and herbs. Beautiful and delicious and very quick to make

-Avocado split! Split open the avocado, remove the seed, and mash the ripe avocado to the desired texture. Top with sliced tomatoes, sea salt, and lime juice for a fast, nutritious breakfast or snack.

NOTES

This way of life is straightforward if you want it to be. Some recipes can be time-consuming, but most alkaline eating is effortless. You will consume many healthy, natural foods with healing powers and beautiful natural tastes enhanced by your creativity. You cannot go wrong if you are using alkaline foods. Here are a few ideas for you to try that you could easily do with little to no prep.

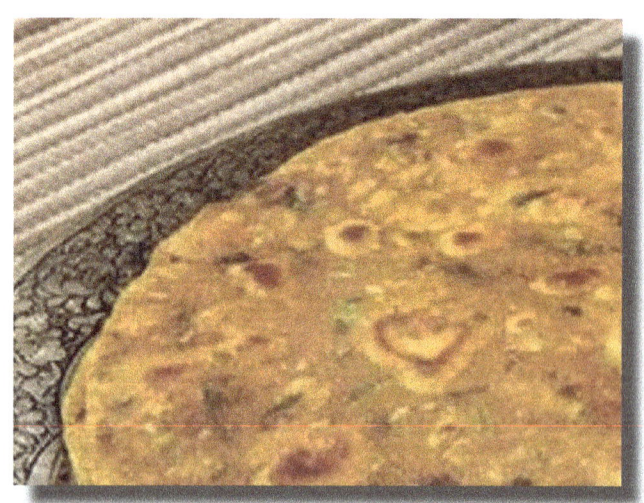

MAPLE MILLET
PORRIDGE

RECIPE 30

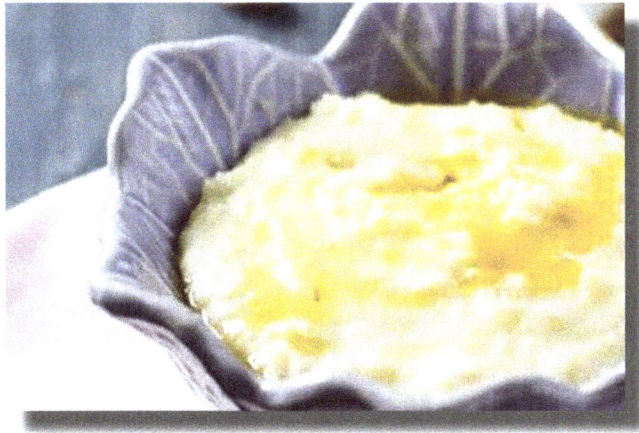

INGREDIENTS

1 cup Millets

4 cups Water

1 pinch Salt

1 tbsp Powder

Maple Syrup to taste

INSTRUCTIONS

1. Boil water in a large pot.

2, Add salt and the millets to the pot.

3. Cover and lower the flame. Cook for 15 minutes.

4. Add cinnamon and almond water.

5. Almond water is made by soaking almonds in water and then blending and straining the mixture to create a creamy, nutty drink. It's often sweetened and flavored with ingredients like vanilla or honey.

6. Continue to cook the millets for 20 minutes.

7. Add some maple syrup and stir. Try to adjust the thickness.

INSTRUCTIONS II

OPTIONS:

TO THICKEN AND ADD FLAVOR

- Mashed ripe bananas can add natural sweetness and thickness to porridge. Mash a ripe banana and stir it into the porridge as it cooks.

- Adding a spoonful of almond, cashew, or tahini (sesame seed butter) to the porridge can add creaminess and thickness.

- Coconut cream is thick and creamy, making it a great addition to porridge. Stir in a tablespoon or two of coconut cream while the porridge cooks.

Your dish is ready!

- Quinoa and Alkaline Veggies! Cook quinoa according to package instructions and mix it with chopped vegetables like bell peppers, mushrooms, tomatoes, cucumbers, and avocado. Drizzle with olive oil, lemon juice, and herbs. Beautiful and delicious and very quick to make

-Avocado split! Split open the avocado, remove the seed, and mash the ripe avocado to the desired texture. Top with sliced tomatoes, sea salt, and lime juice for a fast, nutritious breakfast or snack.

NOTES

As you embark on this journey of self-discovery and wellness, remember that you are enough, just as you are. You deserve all the blessings that life has to offer, including vibrant health and happiness.

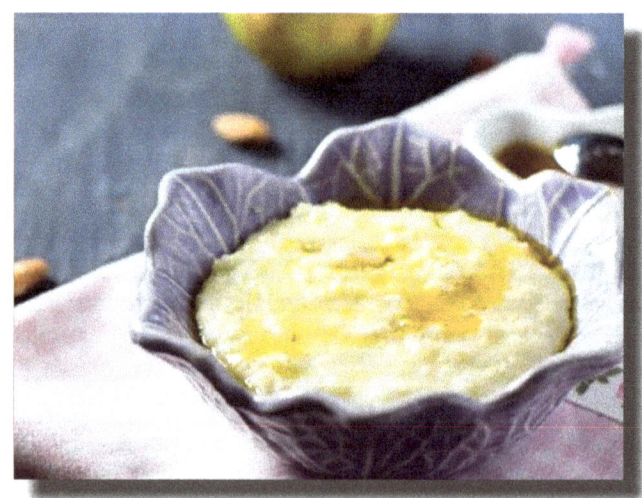

CHICKPEA FRITTATA

RECIPE 31

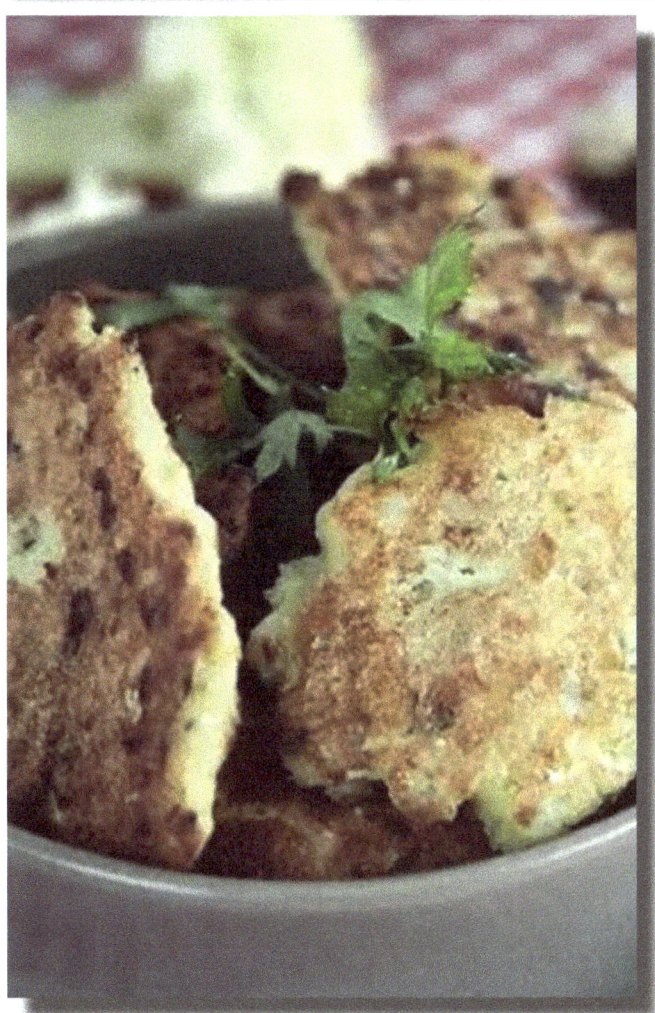

INGREDIENTS

1 cup Chickpea Flour

1 cup Water

1 cup Zucchini, sliced

1/2 cup Chopped Onion

1/2 tsp Black Pepper

4 tbsp Olive Oil

1 clove Garlic, grated

1/2 cup Chopped Spring Onions

Salt to taste

INSTRUCTIONS

1. Preheat the oven to 375F or 190C.

2. Grease a baking pan or tray.

3. Add all ingredients except oil and spring onions in a large bowl.

4. Add 1-2 tablespoons of oil to the large bowl of batter.

5. Add it to the greased pan or tray.

6. Bake for 30-45 minutes.

7. Take it out and slice it into thin slices.

8. Garnish with spring onions and serve.

NOTES

With these alkaline recipes, you nourish not just your body but your spirit as well. You feed your soul with love, kindness, and the purest intentions.

LEAN, GREEN, FENNEL MINT SMOOTHIE

RECIPE 32

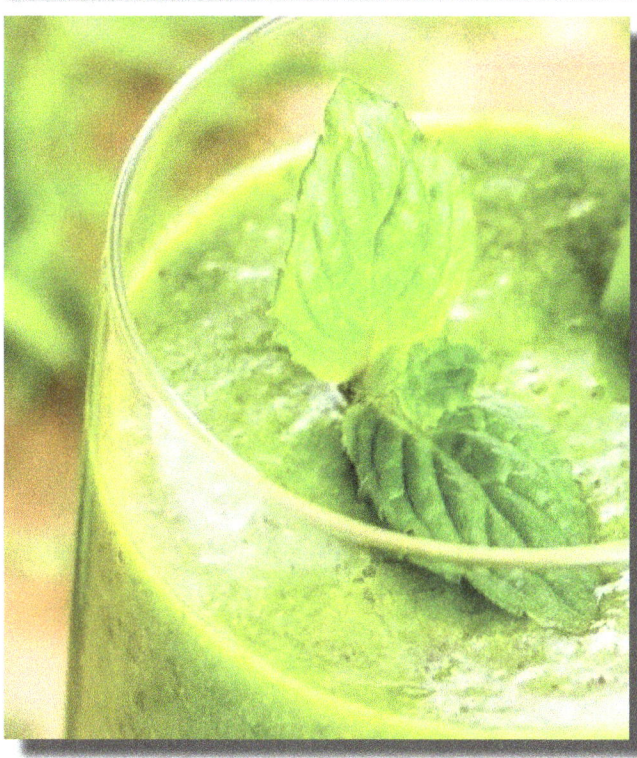

INGREDIENTS

1/2 Cucumber, sliced

2 cups Spinach

1/2 Fennel Bulb

1/4 cup Fresh Mint Leaves

1/2 serves of an Avocado

1 tbsp Chia Seeds*

Protein Powder

1/2 cup Coconut Water (from a young coconut)

1/2 cup Ice

*If possible, soak the chia seeds 10 minutes or overnight before use to enhance the living enzymes and health benefits

NOTES

Your body is a sacred temple that carries you through life's journey. Treat it with the utmost care and respect, and it will reward you with boundless energy, vitality, and joy.

INSTRUCTIONS

1. Add ingredients into a powerful, high-speed blender, and blend until smooth and creamy for ultimate enjoyment!

ALKALINE NOT NACHOS

RECIPE 33

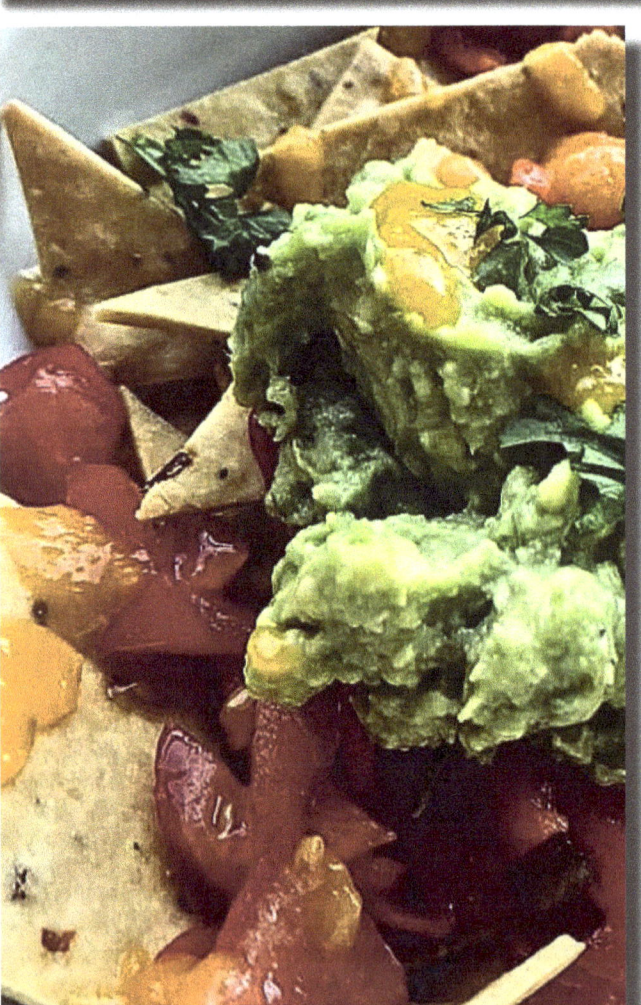

INGREDIENTS

1 bag of alkaline-friendly tortilla chips (look for brands made with spelt or other whole grains)

1 cup cooked black beans, drained and rinsed

1 cup diced tomatoes

1 cup diced bell peppers (any color)

1/2 cup sliced black olives

1/4 cup diced red onion

1/2 cup sliced jalapeños (optional, for heat)

1 cup shredded alkaline-friendly cheese (such as almond or cashew cheese)

1/4 cup chopped fresh cilantro

Lime wedges for serving

Optional toppings: sliced avocado, dairy-free sour cream, salsa, or guacamole

INSTRUCTIONS

1. Preheat Oven: Preheat your oven to 375°F (190°C).

2, Arrange Chips: Spread the alkaline-friendly tortilla chips in a single layer on a large baking sheet.

3. Layer Ingredients: Sprinkle the cooked black beans, diced tomatoes, diced bell peppers, sliced black lives, diced red onion, and sliced jalapeños (if using) evenly over the tortilla chips.

4. Add Cheese: Sprinkle the shredded alkaline-friendly cheese over the nacho toppings.

5. Bake: Place the baking sheet in the oven for 10-15 minutes or until the cheese is melted and bubbly.

6. Garnish: Remove the nachos from the oven and sprinkle chopped fresh cilantro over the top. Serve with lime wedges on the side.

7. Serve: Serve the alkaline nachos hot with your favorite toppings, such as sliced avocado, dairy-free sour cream, salsa, or guacamole.

NOTES

Enjoy these flavorful and satisfying alkaline nachos as a delicious snack or appetizer. Adjust the toppings according to your preferences and dietary needs.

Take time to savor each bite of all your meals. Notice the colors, textures, smells, and flavors of the food on your plate. Chew slowly and pay attention to the sensations of taste and smell as you eat. Eating mindfully can enhance your enjoyment of food and promote better digestion. Be sure to cook with positive energy and gratitude, the positive energy will reflect in your dishes.

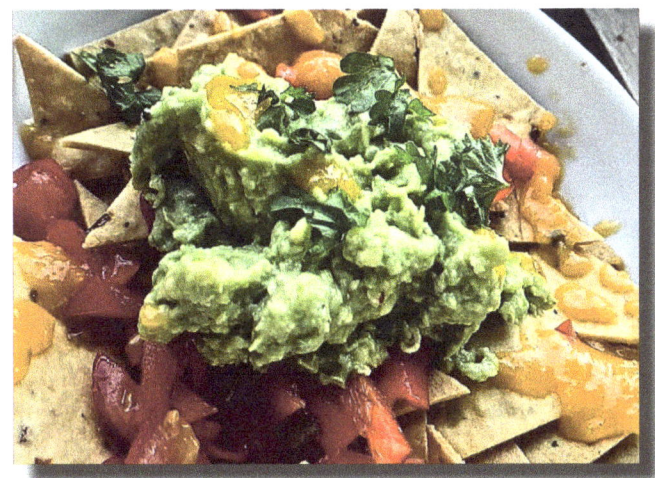

ALKALINE EDAMAME AND MUSHROOM **PASTA**

RECIPE 34

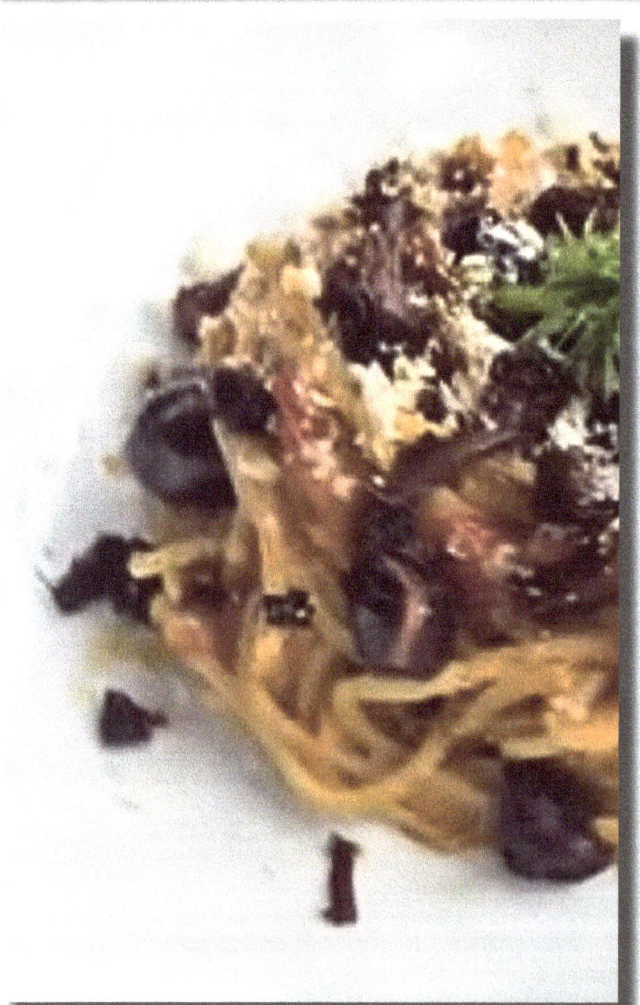

INGREDIENTS

8 oz (about 225g) edamame pasta or spelt pasta

1 cup shelled edamame beans

2 cups sliced mushrooms (button mushrooms, cremini, or shiitake)

2 cloves garlic, minced

2 tablespoons olive oil

1/4 cup vegetable broth

1 teaspoon lemon zest

2 tablespoons lemon juice or lime juice

Salt and pepper to taste

Fresh parsley or basil, chopped, for garnish

Optional: red pepper flakes for heat, nutritional yeast for cheesy flavor

INSTRUCTIONS

1. Cook Pasta: Cook the pasta according to the instructions in a pot of boiling salted water until al dente. Drain and set aside, reserving about 1/2 cup of pasta cooking water.

2. Prepare Edamame and Mushrooms: Heat olive oil over medium heat in a large skillet. Add minced garlic and cook for about 1 minute until fragrant. Add sliced mushrooms and cook for 5-7 minutes until they release moisture and brown.

3. Add Edamame: Stir in shelled edamame beans and cook for an additional 2-3 minutes until they are heated through.

4. Combine Pasta and Vegetables: Add the cooked pasta to the skillet with the mushrooms and edamame. Toss to combine, adding vegetable broth or water as needed to create a sauce that coats the pasta evenly.

5. Stir in lemon zest and lemon juice. Season with salt and pepper to taste. Add red pepper flakes for heat or nutritional yeast for a cheesy flavor if desired.

6. Serve: Divide the pasta into serving bowls. Garnish with chopped fresh parsley or basil for a pop of color and freshness.

7. Enjoy: Serve the alkaline edamame and mushroom pasta hot alongside a fresh green salad or steamed vegetables for a complete and nutritious meal.

NOTES

This alkaline pasta dish is delicious and satisfying. It is packed with protein, fiber, and essential nutrients from edamame, mushrooms, and pasta.

Give yourself a few moments each day to reflect on things you are grateful for. This can be as simple as appreciating the sun's warmth on your skin or the company of a loved one. Cultivating gratitude can shift your perspective and help you focus on the positive aspects of life. You Deserve a Magical Life.

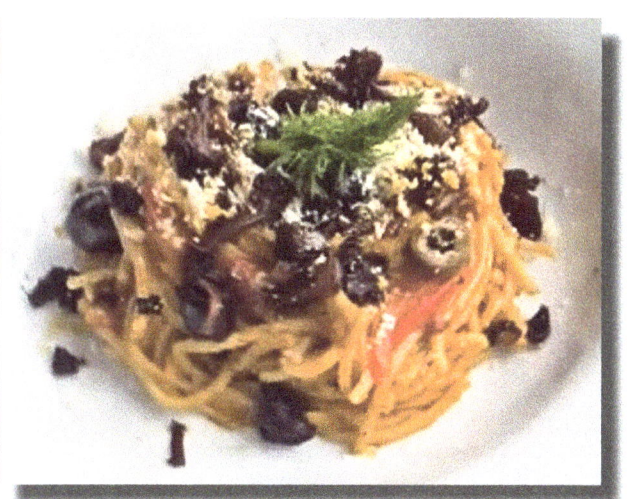

CONCLSION

Alkaline diets promote your overall health in many ways. As modern diets are highly acidic, many nutritionists opt for this diet. Alkaline breakfast recipes are the best way to balance the body's pH levels. French toast, apple pancakes, avocado breakfast salad, mixed sprout salad, and kale chickpea mash are among the best alkaline breakfast recipes. The ingredients used in these recipes are rich in various vitamins and minerals that help boost your health. Hence, try these delicious breakfast recipes and enjoy their benefits.

I leave you with this gentle reminder: within your being lies a reservoir of knowledge, wisdom, and worth beyond measure. You are not merely a vessel for healing but a sacred guardian of your own well-being. As you journey forth with the nourishing recipes and holistic practices shared within these pages, remember that you possess the innate ability to heal, thrive, and reclaim your vitality. Embrace each step of your journey with compassion and gratitude, for every choice you make towards nourishing your body and nurturing your soul, is a testament to your strength and resilience. May you find peace in the journey, wisdom in the challenges, and joy in the healing moments. Remember, you are worthy of love, you are deserving of health, and you have the power to transform your life from within. Trust in your inner wisdom, listen to the whispers of your heart, and may your path be illuminated by the light of self-love and self-care. As you close this chapter and embark on the next, may you always carry this truth in your heart: that you are enough, just as you are, and your journey towards health and healing is a beautiful testament to the power of your spirit.

May you be filled with pride and accomplishment as you prepare each meal. You are a powerful creator, shaping your destiny with every choice.
With love and blessings,
Sheena Marie

NOTES

In your daily life, set aside time each day to write in a journal. Use this time to reflect on your thoughts, feelings, and experiences without judgment. Write down anything that comes to mind, whether it's worries, goals, or moments of joy. Journaling can help you gain insight into your inner world and promote self-awareness.

Author: Sheena Marie

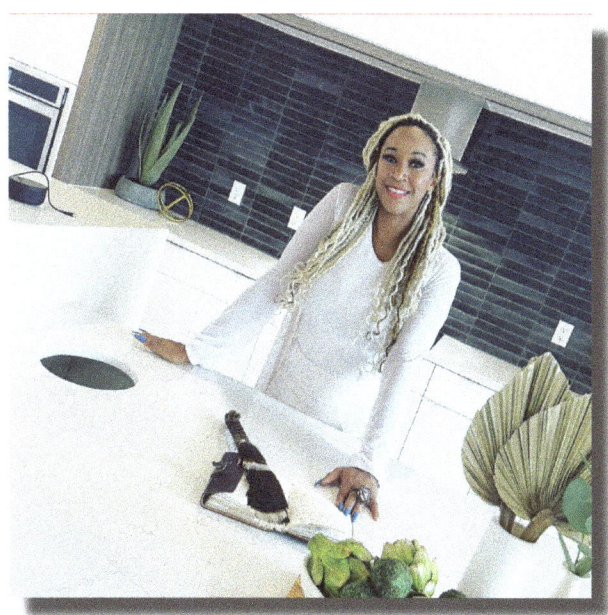

Sheena Marie is a healthcare powerhouse, bringing over fifteen years of enriching experience to the field. Beyond her role as a healthcare professional, she's also known as an Alkaline Chef, elevating the healing power of food to new levels. Sheena is a passionate advocate for total health, encompassing physical, mental, spiritual, emotional, and financial well-being.

Picture yourself at health retreats in the tranquil Usha Village in Honduras—more than just a vacation, it's a transformative journey. Mentored by the legendary Queen Afua, Sheena proudly identifies as a Sacred Woman. Her influence and leadership in the healthcare realm are truly inspiring. Sheena's journey is remarkable, triumphing over cancer and womb issues using her methods. The magic has worked for countless others, propelling her to become a
world-renowned spiritualist and celebrated author.

Sheena Marie is here to guide you towards health and wholeness. Her teachings fuse spirituality with the vibrant goodness of alkaline foods, making the journey as delicious as it is transformative. Prepare to heal your body and elevate your spirit, all under the caring guidance of a true health guru. Your path to becoming one with the Divine has never been more delicious.

www.ingramcontent.com/pod-product-compliance
Lightning Source LLC
Chambersburg PA
CBHW042359070526
44585CB00029B/3000